"With its real-talk conversational tone, *Compared to W*̶̶ woman living in our crazy-making culture of impos̶̶ pursuit of bodily perfection. Despite her claim to exemplify the ordinary, Heather has written a book with the potential to accomplish something truly extraordinary. Comparison is a prison—and the truth within these pages is enough to set captive women free!"

> —**Jena Morrow,** author of *Hollow*

"*Compared to Who?* is a much-needed, gospel-centered approach to the titanic struggle women face when they look in the mirror. Creekmore's voice is refreshingly honest, and she comes alongside the reader as a friend, helping women leave behind the idol of beauty and embrace the outrageous beauty of Jesus. Compelling, well-researched, and a helpful read."

> —**Mary DeMuth,** author of *Worth Living: How God's Wild Love Makes You Worthy*

"If you've ever wanted to find freedom in the body you've been given, this book is for you. Heather takes you by the hand, and with solid biblical principles, exposes the lies about beauty. She'll help you feel differently about the body you have—not the one you *think* you need. You'll find freedom on these pages."

> —**Jennifer Dukes Lee,** author of *The Happiness Dare* and *Love Idol*

"In *Compared to Who?* Heather Creekmore is so real you'll feel like you are having a sleepover with your hilariously honest best friend. By the time you are done with this book, you'll have no excuses left. Ultimately, we all want to feel beautiful, but first we have to decide that we are. This book is a call to a higher level of understanding about our worth, our bodies, and our futures. And if you are as honest as Heather is, you'll be changed for the better—heart, body, and soul."

> —**Jennifer Strickland,** speaker, author of *Beautiful Lies, More Beautiful Than You Know,* and *Girl Perfect,* URMore.org

"Real, raw, relatable, and refreshing. Heather speaks my language. She put words to the very things I and many other women subconsciously do and struggle with. She tells it like it is, cuts out the clichés, and powerfully challenges her reader—all with grace, humor, and Truth. Every woman should read this book!"

> —**Jordan Lee Dooley,** Founder of The SoulScripts, author of *COLLEGE* and *BeLoved*

"Heather Creekmore holds up a biblical mirror for each of us to look into as we battle body image issues. With both humor and camaraderie, this gifted author tenderly unlocks the door to our self-made prison of body hatred. Heather invites us to join her in embracing new levels of freedom from our cycle of chronic comparisons. With concrete questions to think through after each chapter, this book is a must read for anyone who looks at herself and thinks, 'If only . . .' Grab a friend—or your daughter—and let's start a healthy, Christ-centered discussion on both the root of our body image issues and the solution."

> —**Jani Ortlund,** Renewal Ministries

"Heather Creekmore dives into the underbelly of what most women need to hear, and don't hear enough–how our battle isn't with our bodies, but with our hearts. She gently, and often with delightful humor, leads readers into a deeper exploration to find hope and a contentedness with the bodies God created and then encourages us to step out into this world as the beautiful and whole women God meant for us to be. Every woman and young girl should read this book!"

—**Lee Wolfe Blum,** speaker, mental health practitioner, and author of *Table in the Darkness: A Healing Journey Through an Eating Disorder* and *Brave Is the New Beautiful*

"Heather Creekmore gets it. She's compared herself to other women and has felt empty, minimized, and alone. But she's also experienced the power of God to live differently. So if you're ready to finally dig up the deep roots of your own body image issues, Heather is just the right guide to lead you into freedom."

—**Margot Starbuck,** author of *Unsqueezed: Springing Free From Skinny Jeans, Nose Jobs, Highlights, and Stilettos*

"Finally! Someone is tackling this important issue by aiming at the roots. Heather refuses to offer platitudes or quick fixes but instead takes us to the real battle–the one that rages in our hearts. Reading *Compared to Who?* is like sitting down with a wise friend who's determined to see us move toward deeper healing and freedom. This book is both convicting and refreshing."

—**Kendra Dahl,** blogger, Kendradahl.com

"Heather bravely says out loud the embarrassing body shaming thoughts women silently struggle with despite the church's message that we are loved just as we are and society's anthem that every women is beautiful in her own way. With relatable stories, study questions, and Scripture, *Compared to Who?* brings a fresh look at the root of the issue and what the Bible says about finding freedom, once and for all, from the body image battle that plagues our mothers, daughters, and friends."

—**Rachel Randolph,** author of *Nourished: A Search for Health, Happiness, and a Full Night's Sleep*, http://www.thenourishedmama.com/

"As a pastor's wife and women's ministry leader, I've had countless conversations with women about body image and their relationship with food. It is perhaps the most common struggle we have, even among Christian women. That's why I'm grateful for Heather Creekmore's new book, *Compared to Who?*–because the church so desperately needs biblical resources on this issue, and this book is both heart-level and helpful. I will be recommending it to many women."

—**Christine Hoover,** author of *Messy Beautiful Friendship* and *From Good to Grace*

"Heather Creekmore is addressing a significant and important issue that is as old as time. Since Eve, I doubt there has ever been a woman who has been completely content with every aspect of her body. And even Eve, once tempted by what was 'pleasing to the eye' fashioned a fig leaf to cover parts of her body. Indeed, the goal of this important book is to help countless women get back to the 'garden' and stand before the only mirror that really matters: her Creator. And believe God, just like Eve once did, when he says, 'It is good.'"

—**Roland C. Warren,** President/CEO of Care Net and author, *Bad Dads of the Bible*

Compared to Who?

A PROVEN PATH TO IMPROVE YOUR BODY IMAGE

Heather Creekmore

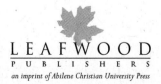

LEAFWOOD
P U B L I S H E R S

an imprint of Abilene Christian University Press

COMPARED TO WHO?

A Proven Path to Improve Your Body Image

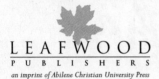

LEAFWOOD
PUBLISHERS
an imprint of Abilene Christian University Press

Published in association with The Gates Group, 1403 Walnut Lane, Louisville, KY 40223.

Cover design by ThinkPen Design, LLC
Interior text design by Sandy Armstrong, Strong Design

Leafwood Publishers is an imprint of Abilene Christian University Press
ACU Box 29138
Abilene, Texas 79699

1-877-816-4455
www.leafwoodpublishers.com

17 18 19 20 21 22 / 7 6 5 4 3 2 1

Acknowledgments

I am so grateful for a community of friends and family who love and encourage me well.

To Eric—Thank you for your unwavering love, support, and belief in me. I'm glad we get to spend the rest of our lives together. I love you very much.

To Zach, Katie, Trevor, and Drew—Thank you for steadfastly remembering to pray for mommy's book during family worship time. I know that some days you've had to wait for your peanut butter and jelly or cereal until I finished a thought, but you've extended much grace to me in that. Thank you for playing LEGOs without fighting and giving me the freedom to write. I love each of you more than you could know.

To Mom and Dad—Thank you for enabling me to pursue my dreams and for your endless love and support. Thank you for communicating your belief that I could do anything I set my mind to. I love you very much and can't aptly communicate the depth of my appreciation for you.

To Lois and Tim—Thank you for caring for our brood through my seasons of writing. Thank you for loving us well. I love and appreciate you both.

Special thanks to the amazing gang of women at our other baby, Mission Church. Thanks especially Laurel Ewing, Jen Bazhaw, Christine Salinas, Brandy Moore, Brandi Webster, Erin Harding, Jennifer Rodriguez (aka J-Rod), and Tricia Vincent. You never got tired of hearing my book-related travails. Your steadfast encouragement—through texts, cards, and conversations—means more than you could know. I love that we get to do life together.

To my other supportive friends (whom I am afraid to name because I'll likely miss someone)—but to Lisa Beegle, Karla Hess, April Birtwistle (aka Birt), Deena Brown, Heidi Hark, Roland and Yvette Warren, Amy Bass, Carissa Bell, and editor extraordinaire, Trisha Mugo. Thank you for your prayers, for reading early rough (and I mean really rough) drafts (and not laughing at me). Thanks for generously agreeing to let me share some of your stories in these pages. And thanks for your encouragement. I love you all dearly, no matter how many miles may separate us.

To the contributors of *Compared to Who?* (the blog): You ladies rock! Thank you for all you've done to help grow the blog and encourage other women. Sharing your personal body image stories has empowered other women to find freedom in this issue. Thank you for all you do!

Special thanks to Don Gates, for not giving up on this project (and for learning more about women's body image issues than he ever imagined he would), and to the great team at Leafwood for making this dream a reality.

Above all, I'd like to thank Jesus for saving me and for graciously showing me the path to true freedom.

Dedication

I sat in our spit-up covered brown leather chair nursing a baby—my fourth baby in as many years—and I said to my husband, "I want to start blogging."

He laughed. Then, when he realized I was serious, he reminded me of our four, nowhere close to self-sufficient children and our even younger church (one we planted six months earlier). "Blogging? Why would you want to do that? Do you really think you have time?"

"Yes! I want to! I really, really want to start writing. I need to start writing."

"Okay, then. Do it!"

To my wonderful husband, Eric,
who likely had no idea what he was agreeing to on that day.
Thank you for your unwavering support of my writing career.
You told me to keep going when I wanted to quit. You bought
me books on becoming a writer. You made me press "send"
when I wasn't sure words sounded good enough. You enabled
me and allowed me to pursue a lifelong dream.
I love you.

Contents

Part One
The Spiritual Root of Our Body Image Issues

Part Two
The Spiritual Solution to Body Image Issues

Introduction

It's the first week of January. You pick the year.

Every. Single. Year.

Turn on your television this early in the month and—unless there's a freak blizzard—I promise you this. The weather will not be the lead news story.

No. First and foremost in every program's lineup will be a segment on how you can improve your body this year. New year, new you! Lose the weight, finally! This is your year!

We eat it up. Maybe this *is* my year!

On one mild January 2, I plopped myself down in front of the *Today Show*. Favorite purple coffee mug in hand, I waited with great anticipation for the special "weight loss and your health" segment to begin.

Oooh . . . what will they tell me? What juicy weight loss or exercise tip will they give to transform my life? Is Paleo still the hottest diet, or should I follow something better now? Are carbs bad and eggs good now? Or do I have that backward?

A surge of excitement rushed through me. Maybe it was just the coffee.

Back from the commercial break, the segment began.

"Kids, keep it down." I yelled. "Mommy needs to hear this! *Quiet!*"

Volume up. I settle in. Nice anchor banter. Hmm . . . cute dress. Good to see you, too.

Yeah, yeah, yeah. Enough with the small talk. Get to the good stuff. Some child will need a drink refill or a potty trip soon. I don't have all day here, people. Spill the hot secrets already.

"So, what should we do to meet our weight loss or health goals this year?" The smiling host tossed the question to her guest like a hot potato. *Finally!*

Here it comes. This is going be good. Where's my pen?

"Well, Savannah, the number one thing that people can do this year if they want to lose weight is to watch what they eat. If they consume only healthy, highly nutritious foods and then add some exercise to their daily routines—those unwanted pounds will melt off."

Are you kidding me? Did she really just say to eat right and exercise?

Wonk. Wonk. Wonk.

What's Your Story?

I know we just met and all, but I need to confess something. I struggled with my body image most of my life. And I tried just about everything out there that I could think of, find, or afford to change it.

Nothing ever worked.

Until recently, that is, when God took me on a journey through my body image challenges and showed me (in ways that I never expected) how I could find true freedom and healing.

But, unlike the hype and letdown of a January 2 news story, I hope to offer you something unexpected in the pages that follow. In fact, my goal is to completely change your perspective on the whole body image issue—in ways you'd never even guess! I'm not going to just tell you, "It's what's on the inside that counts." (This is, to me, the Christian equivalent of "eat right and exercise.") Instead, I want to motivate you to pursue a fresh level of freedom that stale clichés could never inspire.

I weave my story into this book. I'll just be real—it's not amazing. I've never been a supermodel. (Or even an average model—although at age eighteen I *did* get to wear a shiny beige pantsuit for a small-town Chamber of Commerce fashion show. *Yeah, it was kind of a big deal.*)

My tale exemplifies the ordinary. But for that reason, I hope you can relate. It's the testimony of how God helped me—a "normal" girl—who believed (sometimes obsessively) that her life would be better if only she were more beautiful.

When I write it out like that, it sounds a little silly. How shallow of me, right? (I'm turning pink from embarrassment as I type.) Yet, it's true. My thought life should have centralized around endeavors with greater meaning, but instead I spent a lot of my mental energy and time pursuing a better body. If I could just be thinner, then I could be happy—or so I believed.

Perhaps the same holds true for you. Maybe you know you struggle. Or maybe you've never admitted to anyone that your thought life orbits planets of worry over your size, shape, or appearance. It's possible that you know you wrestle discontentment with the mirror but never knew what to call it.

Here we'll call it body image. This will be a safe space for us to talk about it—the good, the bad, and the "I can't believe anyone else does or thinks that"—openly. Statistics show that most women engage in an internal war in this arena. If those stats are true, then there's a good chance you struggle, too. I want you to know you have a friend right here who understands that battle. That's also how I hope you'll read this book—like advice from a friend who's been there and is navigating her way out.

If you are weighed down with insecurity or feeling not good enough, or if your negative body image plagues you and impacts your ability to find peace and joy in other areas of this life, I pray God will use this book to reveal his rescue plan for you.

There is hope for victory in your personal battle to be beautiful. Your journey starts here when you ask this question: Compared to who?

Part One

The Spiritual Root

of Our
Body
Image
Issues

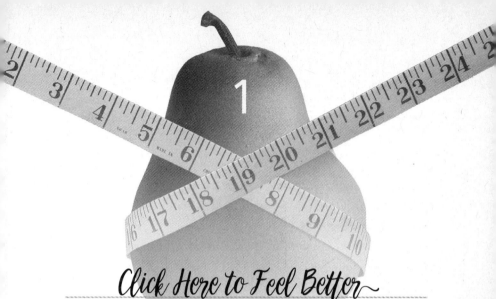

Click Here to Feel Better

"Beauty does not make you happy. A size two does not solve your insecurity. The prettiest clothes and the shiniest hair in the nation is not the combination you need to stop being consumed with how you look. In fact, just the opposite may be true."

—CAMERON RUSSELL, Victoria's Secret Model

Thigh dimples. Belly pooch. Saggy breasts. Stretch marks.

I love to see them.

No. Not on my own body. Yikes! Of course not. That would be silly.

I mean, I have them. We all do. Okay, *most* of us over the age of nineteen bear at least one of these signs of fallen humanity. There are a few fortunate ones out there. But gravity will find them, too. Eventually. It *always* wins.

There is one place where cellulite, love handles, and flab look fantastic. That's on the body of a celebrity.

The better she appears on screen, the more so-called imperfections I want to see.

Click here to see her ugly beach photos.
Click here to see the unedited photo.
Click here to see what she really looked like after she gave birth.
Click here to see her without her makeup.

Sure. Why not? Tabloids and gossip sites happily give us what we want—blown-up photos of celebrity flaws circled in red ink like missed answers on a test.

Did you ever wonder why we like to see them? Why we're happy to look at another woman's so-called body defects?

I have a theory.

I think it's because cellulite, deflated bosoms, and other flaws on the allegedly flawless affirm the average woman's existence. Or, mine at least.

That is, they *seem* to. I expected clicking on those "average" photos would help my problem—make me feel better.

Now my perspective has changed.

Supermodel Letdown

During my formative years, our culture decided to set apart certain female specimens as emblems of beauty. This league of women stood out above all the rest. (Literally, not only were they taller than the average girl, but they also had long legs and minimal body fat, allowing them to appear to tower over us all.) These ladies weren't just models, but supermodels.

"Oh how wonderful it would be to look like that!" So the teenage me thought. It's been a few decades, so I'd be hard-pressed to name too many of them now, but one name I'll never forget is Cindy Crawford. I admired Cindy because, in an era where it seemed like being blonde meant being beautiful, she had brown hair.

And so did I. (Until I figured out how to color it, at least.) She also had a mole. That little brown dot on her face didn't seem to bother her a bit. Yet I had a mole about the same size on my wrist that I obsessed over. Cindy gave me hope. Maybe, someday, my mole could symbolize hotness, too. *If only I could find a way to look more like Cindy Crawford . . .*

Fast-forward a few decades to last month. I sat at my computer scrolling through Facebook when an intriguing photo of my former idol floated by. The picture showed what looked like an unretouched image of Cindy wearing black lingerie, a boa, and a magician-caliber top hat—a recent magazine cover that never made it to the editing department. In it, the supermodel appeared with belly flab, cellulite, and stretch marks. Her untoned thighs looked as dimply as mine. *Were they touching in the middle?* Her stomach bore the marks of pregnancies and age. *I guess my stomach is okay if that's how Cindy's looks! Fabulous!*

Cindy Crawford's cellulite made my day.

I watched as the photo received an abundance of social media attention. (I blog about body image. This wasn't lame. I prefer to call it research.) More viral than the swine flu, millions shared the imperfect cover photo and applauded Cindy.

"What courage she has to let us see that she's real!" some said.

"She's still gorgeous, but now we can all feel a little better about our normalness," others commented.

"She did it on purpose," they speculated. "She wants to be a help for all those struggling with the way they look!"

The supermodel offered a lifeline to the wave of women engulfed in negative body image and everyone cheered.

Until her husband got romantic.

Cindy's husband, Rande Gerber, posted a picture of his love lying by the pool in an orange bikini. He captioned it: "She got flowers and I got her."

So sweet.

Except for one little detail. His Instagram post looked nothing like the leaked *Marie Claire* flabby photo from a few days earlier. There was no sign of stretched skin or dimpled flesh on that forty-nine-year-old's body.

What?

Those other photos, it turns out, were fake. Someone air-brushed Cindy's body to look more regular—a cruel joke on those of us who seek affirmation from flabby celebrity photos.[1]

Cindy Crawford just may have a perfect body. (Or a talented plastic surgeon . . .) Comparison bites us in the cellulite. Again.

Compared to Who?

Can we just be honest? Even when real, those celebrity cellulite photos never actually satisfy. They draw you in; you look, and you seem to feel better for a few minutes. But, like searching for comfort in chocolate chip cookie dough, an hour later your stomach aches.

That gut-level unrest—that's called comparison. And comparison cures nothing.

When you feel comparison surge inside, you better cue the *Jaws* music. Nuh-nah, nuh-nah, nuh-nah, nuh-nah. . . . Comparison plays nice at first. "Hey, you are doing just fine." (The music gets louder.) She lets us swim in contentment. (The music gets even louder.) Then, all of a sudden, boom! She finds someone doing "better," shows us how we don't measure up, and yanks us under-water like a shark going for the kill. Her bite leaves a mark, and she drowns us in shame.

Comparison hurts—it hurts our relationships, our children, our marriages, and (most of all) it hurts us. Comparison distracts us from our purpose while keeping us entangled in its petty contests.

I never thought I'd write a book on this topic. Comparison's the one voice in your head you don't want *anyone* to hear. I'm thankful that only God has the superpower of reading our minds.

I'd rather no one knew about the times I wondered if I wore a larger or smaller clothing size than someone else. I'd rather no one heard how my brain analyzed her hair, or her clothing, or her shape, or her skin, and then compared it to my own.

That stuff is private. And kind of embarrassing.

Confessions of a Chronic Comparer

Motherhood introduced me to a brand-new realm of comparison. Admittedly, I compared myself to the other women around me long before a baby boarded my belly, but once I was with child, the opportunities to compare multiplied.

I compared my weight gain to that of every other pregnant woman I knew, saw on TV, read about in a magazine, or heard someone else talk about. Sure, I understood it was healthy to gain, but deep down I wanted to know where I stood in my own imaginary competition where the skinniest pregnant woman wins. I compared others' custom nursery themes to my "nursery in a bag" set from the Target clearance rack. I compared what strollers they bought, what birthing classes they took, and the cuteness of their maternity wardrobe. I thought pregnancy made me tired but, seriously, all that comparison proved just as exhausting.

The baby arrived. Soon, keeping up in the game became even more complicated. Like a sponge, I absorbed every nugget of hearsay data on how other babies progressed. *Her baby slept through the night. Her baby ate on a perfect schedule. Her baby sang the alphabet song—at nine months old!* Consumed with where my little guy fit into the mix, I panicked. He hadn't smiled. He hadn't rolled over. Sleeping, yeah, that wasn't happening.

Would he be slow? Was there a problem? Was I doing something wrong? Or, worse, was I just a bad mom *(already!)?* If comparison was a disease, I suffered chronically. I needed to stop, but I didn't know how.

The mommy comparison game is rough, but it's not the worst. Of the many ways women can—and do—compare themselves, it's the physical comparisons that can cause the most damage. When we look at another woman's body, compare it to our own, and then decide that having a different build, hair, height, or weight would somehow be better, an internal war begins—a fight with our body image.

My friend Sydney said she first felt the shark bite of comparison at six years old. She noticed her friend's legs were skinny, while hers were thick and muscular. From there, her battle escalated. She fought condemnation. "You should look better, eat better, and exercise more . . ." echoed in her head all through her teen years. Shame told her she was unacceptable and that she'd have a hard time finding a boyfriend or a husband with legs like that.

Can I tell you something difficult? If you saw a picture of Sydney, you wouldn't think her legs were large. At all. Sydney's problem was with her body image—not with her body.

I've struggled in the same ways. In fact, I hesitate to share with you the depths of my depravity in the body image arena. Disordered eating, weight obsession, exercise dependency, and insecurity—I wrestled them all. Satan told me the same lie he told Sydney—that my legs were too big. And that one thought ignited a firestorm of body image issues that continued for decades.

I am frightened for you to know the details of my struggle, like the fact I still sometimes hide candy wrappers in the trash can instead of placing them on the top. It might disturb you to know how badly I wished I could throw up after binge eating. You may be turned off to hear that I fight hard not to walk into a room full of women and mentally divide them into two categories: thinner than me and not thinner than me. I share my secrets not to humiliate myself, but with the hope that my honesty will help others know they aren't alone. Because, truth is, those of us who struggle often feel like we are the only ones trapped in the crazy land of body worry. For that reason, few talk about it.

I find it hard to talk about sometimes, too. Writing seems easier, so I started a blog. I found the more I wrote about my personal struggle, the more emails I would receive that said, "Thank you. I thought I was the only one who had thoughts like this!" Eventually, I titled my blog *Compared to Who?* (For all of my badge-carrying friends in the grammar police, I know you'd rather it read *Compared to Whom?* I'm sorry. It just sounded too uppity!) As I began to write more on the topic and speak with women about body image issues directly, I noticed a common theme—their body image struggles seemed to stem from comparison's bite.

Comparison Is "Abs"solutely Silly

Comparison lies to us. It never regards the truth. It leaves out important details about age, lifestyle, genetics, ethnicity, and, oh, like a million other important factors when it tells us we should look different. I think of a woman I met through the blog last year named Whitney. She's ethnically, genetically, and regionally (she lives in the Northeast) predisposed to having pale skin. Yet comparison sneaked in and whispered, "You aren't beautiful. You are too white—like Casper, the friendly ghost. That's ugly."

I've also brawled against comparison's ridiculous jabs. Many other women do, too. I know this because some women lack a filter between their mind and their mouth and have clued me in to the (otherwise secret) struggle.

It happened as I waited for my daughter's dance class to finish. Moms aren't actually allowed in the dance studio because, here in Texas, we take our kindergarteners' extracurricular activities very seriously. Having moms inside the classes would be dangerous. (Think: Lifetime Channel's *Dance Moms*.) So, instead, we sit in this small waiting room during the forty-five-minute class and, because making conversation is so 1997, everyone stares at their phones.

Right before class ended, the studio door opened. Every head popped up from its screen-slumped position, expecting to see a line of six-year-olds exit the room. But instead, an older girl—one of the dance studio's helpers—walked out and closed the studio door behind her. As this lone girl maneuvered her way through the gaggle of waiting moms, she got a few stares. She wore a bright, sports bra-type tank top and black spandex dance shorts. She had a cute little body for a soon-to-be preteen, and everyone noticed.

Or at least one woman did.

The front door had barely shut behind her when one of the moms (the one without a filter) loudly asked the crowd, "Did you *see* her abs?" We all had. Her sculpted core looked magazine perfect. But she was barely ten. Her skin had never stretched so that her entire abdominal region could reorganize to accommodate a growing baby (or four in my case). We were a group of moms and this girl, she had likely just finished the third grade! *The third grade!*

No one responded.

So this mom (who obviously worked out and was some sort of abs aficionado) just kept talking.

"Wow, I wish my stomach looked like that."

Crickets.

Then she involved her own little girl, whom I guessed to be about five years old. While patting her daughter's belly, she made the following statement about the child: "She doesn't have any abs at all."

Too stunned to say anything, I stared at her blankly. At least, I hope my expression appeared blank and didn't reveal what I really thought. *Did a grown woman really just covet a ten-year-old's abdominal muscles out loud?* She first compared her body (a full-grown woman who carried and birthed the child she had in tow) with that of a pre-tween girl. Then, she taught her daughter how to do the same (with an appropriate amount of dissatisfaction).

Comparison. It's silly.

Chapter Mirror

Watch this video message from Heather for extra encouragement as you dive into this book: http://comparedtowho.me/more -encouragement

Note

[1] Elizabeth Vanmetre, "Cindy Crawford's Leaked Un-Retouched Photos Are Fake, According to Photographer," *Daily News*, March 2, 2015, www .nydailynews.com/entertainment/gossip/cindy-crawford-leaked-photos -fake-photogr-article-1.2134876.

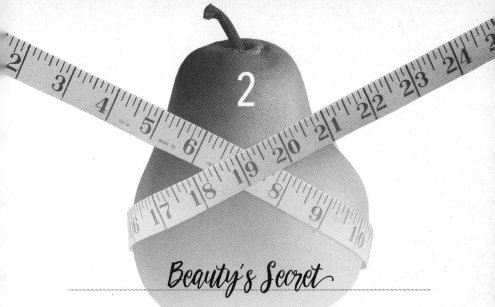

2

Beauty's Secret

"How about now? Am I good enough?
How about now? Will I ever be enough?
If I change, would I find love?"

—Veridia, "Pretty Lies"

Statistics reveal up to 91 percent of women wrestle with body image and either diet or engage in other activities to try to change the way their bodies look.[1]

Did you catch that number—91 percent? Yikes!

Surely, surely, the numbers would be better for Christian women. We love Jesus more than Spanx, right? I figured they'd still be high, but in the mid-eighties, tops.

So I embraced my nerdy side and conducted my own study. Though my research methods may not win national acclaim, my nationwide survey received more than six hundred responses and showed that many women who identified themselves as Jesus-followers still fought negative body image. In truth, the numbers for this segment of the population were just as high, if not a little higher, than the general population.[2]

What? Seems the shark of comparison is eating Christian women alive, too.

So how do we stop it? Can we win our body image battles?

I think so, but the battle is real—and more complex in nature than our clichés accommodate.

Clichés and Zit Creams

"Just stop comparing," some leaders preach. Remember that envy green looks bad on all skin tones and get over it. "Be happy for the other person!" and train your brain with positivity. For almost thirty years, I battled and couldn't find a way to "just stop." Neither mind games nor the affirmation of others freed me. I didn't know how to end comparison's grip.

Intellectually, I knew God loved me, and he valued my insides more than my outsides. But I didn't know how to believe it in a way that rid my worry over what I saw in the mirror. I read all about "true beauty" and yet still cared more about my jeans' size than my prayer time. I heard, "Every woman is beautiful in her own way" and thought: I don't want to be beautiful in my own way, I want to be beautiful like her!

These clichés were as ineffective as using an over-the-counter zit cream on a monster-sized pimple. Allow me to explain.

I've had my fair share of pimples. Through the years, I bought about every product ever advertised to eliminate them. Now that I'm older and have done more research, I see the truth. The real problem that causes the blemish often lurks below the surface. You can use the topical ointments, scrubs, and special soaps, yet most of the time, acne's root is internal—it's systemic.

Even though I could disguise my blemishes with yellow-tinted concealer, and a healthy amount of a thick foundation, they were still under there. They didn't go away just because I dabbed on benzoyl peroxide and made them less noticeable.

This is how I feel about the clichés our culture and even the church use to try to help women with serious body image struggles. They hand over a tube of concealer and a bottle of flesh-colored makeup and claim it's the antidote. "Here, honey, you'll be fine. Just remember, it's what's on the inside that counts."

When I speak to women's groups on this topic, I start with some fun exercises to establish how many of the women in the room wish they could change the way their bodies look.

After we find common ground and acknowledge that almost every woman in the room struggles with her body image and comparison—at some level—I ask this question: "How many of you know it's what's on the inside that counts?"

Every woman in the room raises her hand.

Then I say, "Hey, well, maybe you haven't heard this one. How many of you know that God made every woman beautiful in her own way?"

Again, each hand goes up. Not a single face looks at all surprised or encouraged by this statement.

And then I ask this, "Do you know why these statements don't help?"

They don't.

I didn't, either. I wanted them to work. I knew the Bible. I remembered the story of David and how the Bible says God chose David as the next king of Israel and paid no attention to his outward form (1 Sam. 16:7). He looked only at his heart. I genuinely appreciated this attribute of God . . . while still praying that he would, somehow, make me more physically beautiful.

I won't waste pages belaboring the fact that your greatest beauty lies underneath your skin. Yes, it's true, but I want to give you fresh answers. Here, we're going to find and eliminate the root of your body image battle to transform the way you view your body image to help you find real freedom.

These clichés aren't bad, but they fail to persuade us because they only speak to the surface of our body image struggles, not the root. They add a dab of Zapzyt, but they don't get rid of the pimple.

We Wrestle Not against Cindy Crawford

I've worked for over a decade in the fitness industry. I'm also a pastor's wife and a mommy blogger, so I talk to women on this issue in many different types of environments. I've found that the problem is often the same. Many women believe the core of their problem is what they see in the mirror. They engage in a battle against their physical bodies because they assume if they can change their appearance, they can beat comparison and overcome their body image battle.

Waging battle armed with a straightening iron, toning cream, "war paint" (aka makeup), diet books, and a personal trainer, women believe they'll win the fight. Yet it never works. Our battle isn't with our bodies; it's inside our hearts.

And our real battle isn't even one against comparison or body image—it's against beauty.

Now, please don't misunderstand me. I don't mean our battle is against beautiful women (like Cindy Crawford) or against Photoshop ninjas who alter pictures and make every woman look impossibly good (or not so good in Cindy's case, I guess). Despising Hollywood for making the standards too high or hating the magazine industry for perpetuating those silly standards of beauty would be futile.

Even if Congress banned photo touch-ups, forced every female screen star to fire her stylist and put on twenty pounds, and required our daughters to play with plastic dolls designed with muffin tops and double chins, we would still struggle. It's not the standard of beauty that's the problem. It's beauty, herself—when we idolize beauty. You see, the beauty idol deceives us. It dangles a prize in a beautiful package (picture a Tiffany box) and tells us we can have it as soon as we shape up. Its offer entices. It says beauty will make our lives better.

Beauty tells the mother of two that she would be happier with a ten-year-old's abs. Beauty tells the six-year-old girl that she needs thinner legs to be accepted. Beauty shouts that our marriage, work, friendships, and life in general would be easier if we just looked prettier.

Beauty may tell you that you'd have a husband (or a better one!), a better sex life, more friends, or a higher-paying job if you just chased it a little harder. But, whatever it says, know this. Beauty lies. It points out our destination and then puts us on a treadmill to get there.

Societies have long held their own standards of beauty. Even in ancient times, some women met that standard and others did not. The Bible doesn't shy away from telling us some women were considered beautiful (Rachel) while others weren't (Leah) (Gen. 29:17). I never understood how God could make that distinction between these two sisters. How could he point out that one woman radiated hotness while the other looked better with a veil on? Didn't he know that he made *all* women beautiful? Where was the footnote in my Bible that said Leah had dim eyes but great thighs?

And then I realized something. It's okay for God to point out that some women have great physical beauty and others don't because he knows the truth about beauty. The beauty God designed and the idol of beauty worshipped by our culture are not one and the same. (Alas, I promised not to write about true beauty . . .)

Have you ever wondered why we have such a hard time with beauty? Why we place so much importance on it? It's because we believe beauty's lies. We believe in beauty's ability to deliver on her promises. That's why we must start fighting this beauty battle for what it is, my friend. It looks like a physical fight, but it's really a spiritual battle (Eph. 6:12).

It's (Totally) Rigged

There's a sign by the front door of the gym where I work that says, "Five Reasons to Work Out." Number one reads: No more body image problems.

That's a myth.

I get it. Changing your body seems like the obvious solution to a body image struggle. Yet when you try to battle beauty on her terms, it never works. You can't win. Culture's standards of beauty keep changing. And, even if you reach them, you'll find beauty didn't give you what it promised.

This "I'll never win" feeling escalated for me as I engaged in my personal beauty battle. The game felt rigged—like the carnival balloon pop. Remember that game? So many half-blown-up balloons filled the board that it looked impossible to miss. If I could just throw the dart right at the center of one balloon, surely it would pop. I'd hit it, and nothing would happen. I could hit it again and again, dead-on, a little harder, a little lighter. Yet none of those balloons were ever going to burst.

I could see the right number on the scale. No satisfaction. I could get my hair as straight as a celebrity's. No pop of eternal joy. I could finally have clear skin, a good hair day, and the right outfit on, and still feel like I missed beauty's mark. Despite pouring plenty of dollars and hours into the beauty game, I could not win. (Nor did I ever get to pick out the oversized stuffed animal of my choice!)

Trying to beat beauty? That's impossible. Like a boxer, you may win a few rounds. You may experience weeks when you feel like the prettiest woman in your office or days, like your wedding day, when you know you are the sparkliest gem in the case. But if approached as a competition, your winning streak will come to an end. The new intern they hire will be twenty-one and cover-model gorgeous. Your wedding makeup will wash off. And that white dress? Let's be real. You may never, ever, get that baby zipped up again.

Beauty neither solves our problems nor gives us what we hope. Consider this:

- You can get into the best shape of your life with buns of steel and six-pack abs and still struggle in your marriage (or struggle to find a boyfriend!).
- You can get that long-awaited nose job (the one that will forever change the way you feel about yourself in photographs!) and still not find the joy you desperately desire.
- You could look like a Barbie doll. Your chest can be full, your waist small, and your complexion so flawless it looks airbrushed, but your friends may still betray you.
- You could meet society's standard of beauty and still feel completely insecure about your body.

Getting Off the Treadmill

I want us to get off the treadmill. Not literally, of course—treadmills are fine. (If you like running in place and getting shin splints.)

Webster's Dictionary defines body image as your own mental picture of what your body looks like. In other words, it's what you think about the way you look. Most of our problems have nothing to do with the reality of how our bodies look. Rather, it comes down to how we feel about them, what we think about them. These thoughts and feelings drive us toward certain actions (like dieting, plastic surgery, eating disorders, and addictions). Social scientists classify these actions as resulting from our body image.

In my experience, negative body image tops the list of obstacles women face, and it prevents us from finding true freedom and joy in this life. Comparison gloms on to our body image struggles and imprisons us. Though sometimes it's hard to discern which came first, the comparison or the body image issues, it doesn't really matter. The root of both issues is the same. That's why, for the next several chapters, we'll talk less about comparison directly and focus more on the topic of body image.

When I speak, travel, or just get on Facebook, I often see Christian women stifled from their God-given calling because they don't feel good enough about their bodies to accomplish their purpose. I believe that just as the enemy of our soul, Satan, uses pornography to cripple and bind men, he uses the body image issue to destroy women. If you think that's too strong a statement, I invite you to think with me about what we women do when we battle body image.

- We surrender ourselves to early and extramarital sexual activity because we so desperately seek body affirmation.
- We struggle to engage in meaningful and necessary relationships with other women because we compete with and compare ourselves to them.
- We flounder to find fulfillment in our marriages because we are too insecure to offer our physical bodies as gifts to our husbands.
- We're driven to work *way* more than necessary because we "need" the extra money to have closets full of clothing, drawers full of cosmetics and anti-aging potions, and tanning packages, gym memberships, and spa treatments.

Don't get me wrong. I'm not against a good pedicure (I could use one right now!). If you don't join the gym, I lose my part-time job. But our priorities are out of whack when tanning sessions (or you name the ritual) are no longer luxuries but are necessary for us to feel comfortable going out in public. I recently even had a woman tell me she thought she was too fat to go to church! (I can assure you her problem was not physical.)

When we lack money to tithe or time to serve in a local congregation, but we have a personal trainer and a closet full of designer jeans—something is wrong.

Beauty wins.

Happiness Doesn't Come with Thin Thighs

If you aren't one of the millions of people who watched Victoria's Secret model Cameron Russell's ten-minute TED talk, then allow me to bring you up to speed. TED is a conference devoted to idea sharing. In short—often ten minutes or less—speeches, different influential people share ideas on different topics. Cameron Russell's talk shocked many because she revealed something. She's insecure.

She's an underwear model. During her talk, Cameron looks gorgeous, the envy of women worldwide. Yet she tells young girls not to aspire to be like her. She tells them to "find something more important to do," when they ask about how they could become a model.

And she makes the following statement:

(Most people think) [i]f you are a little bit skinnier and have shinier hair, you will be so happy and fabulous . . . but . . . the thing we never say on camera is: I am insecure. I am insecure because I have to think about what I look like on camera every day. If you are ever wondering, "If I have thinner thighs and shinier hair will I be happier?" You just need to meet a group of models because they have the thinnest thighs and the shiniest hair and the coolest clothes, and they are the most physically insecure women on the planet.

She continues:

> Beauty does not make you happy. A size two does not
> solve your insecurity. The prettiest clothes and the shin-
> iest hair in the nation is not the combination you need
> to stop being consumed with how you look. In fact, just
> the opposite may be true.[3]

Cameron Russell bravely exposes beauty's lie. Yet I wonder how many of the women who viewed this talk believed her. The lie is very, very convincing, and the liar excels at deception.

Here's the good news. Much of our struggle, once we identify it, can be redeemed. You can have hope that someday, soon even, you can and will feel differently about your body. And that one day—soon, I pray—you'll no longer be stuck in the rut of comparing yourself to other women.

I want to help you embark on a journey that I've been on for the past several years. Consider me a sojourner. It would be disingenuous of me to say that I've arrived. Every once in a while, I still hear the *Jaws* music and feel tempted to compare myself to other women. But now I'm better equipped to recognize it and turn it off before the shark attacks. It's not a "fun ship" cruise, necessarily. But if you've been hunkered down in a beauty battleship for a good part of your life—I believe (and pray) the voyage will transform you.

Through the next several chapters, I will share how our hearts deceive us into believing the beauty-equals-happiness lie. We'll start by breaking down the truth about self-esteem and all that culture tells us we need so we can overcome our body image struggles. Then I'll tell you the story of my personal battle with weight and appearance—how I tried to find joy anywhere and everywhere but where it can truly be found.

Then, for the remainder of the book, we'll dig deep into the five steps. These are five general things to do—though each chapter is filled with more specific suggestions—to challenge what you believe about yourself, others, the Bible, and even God. We'll talk about comparison, about changing our habits, about living in community, and about the connection between salvation and our body image issues. Through these pages, I want to inspire you to view your body image battle with a fresh perspective, so you can find the true joy, peace, and freedom that only Jesus offers.

At the end of each chapter that follows, you'll find a Chapter Mirror, a summary of the chapter's main ideas, followed by a set of Heart Exercises for personal or group study. These questions will help you process the material to jump-start your personal transformation.

Psalm 119:11 encourages us to hide God's Word in our hearts so we can avoid the ensnarement of sin. That's why I include a memory verse at the end of each chapter. You may choose to go through these exercises alone or in community with a few friends who also struggle. I highly encourage you to do both. Read through and answer the questions alone first, and then invite a group of women to go through the book again with you. As you'll read in Chapter Ten, community is going to be key to your long-term success in winning this battle against your body image.

I also invite you to become a part of our community on my blog, *Compared to Who?* (comparedtowho.me) and to subscribe to twice weekly encouragement from the site as you go through this process. While there, join me on social media, too, so you know you'll have something positive waiting in your newsfeed to combat all those body image messages that try to tear you down and impede your progress.

Now, if you're ready. Let's get this journey started.

Bon voyage.

Chapter Mirror

Though comparison pretends to offer hope for our body image problems, she's more like a shark that attacks and wounds us. The root of our body image and comparison struggles is the same—a battle against beauty and beauty's lies. It is an internal battle, not an external one. Our struggles are spiritual in nature—a fight that takes place in our hearts—not on our bodies.

Heart Exercises

Today, I want to encourage you to get real about your body image struggle. Read Genesis 1:27, 2:21–25 and all of Genesis 3 and answer the following questions.

1. From this passage, what do we learn about the way God created us?

2. Shame didn't exist until Genesis 3, when sin entered the world. What can we observe about the way Adam and Eve's sin impacted how they viewed their physical bodies? Did they need God to tell them they were naked, or was their new awareness a direct result of their sin?

3. If women have been hiding their bodies since creation, what does that tell us about our struggle with body image?

4. In what ways did you previously view your struggle as an external problem? How likely are you to compare yourselves to others?

5. Read Genesis 29:17. Do you think it's okay for God's Word to tell us that Rachel was more physically beautiful than Leah? Why?

6. What is your hope for this so-called voyage? Do you desire freedom in this area of your life?

7. Optional: Today, make a vow to not give up on this journey to find body image freedom. Using the hashtag #ComparedtoWho, write one sentence about how you hope to change through this process, and post it on social media as a marker that today your steps toward body image freedom begin. Or, if you aren't a social media person, mark the date on your calendar or in your journal along with your objective.

I want to see myself as a whole person – in God's image – not just the sum of my body parts. 3/21/22

Memory verse: "Lead me in the path of your commandments, for I delight in it. Incline my heart to your testimonies, and not to selfish gain! Turn my eyes from looking at worthless things; and give me life in your ways" (Ps. 119:35–37).

Notes

[1] "11 Facts about Body Image," DoSomething.org, accessed May 1, 2014, https://www.dosomething.org/facts/11-facts-about-body-image.

[2] Heather Creekmore, "National Study of Christian Women and Body Image," press release, *Compared to Who?* (blog), conducted in April 2014, http://comparedtowho.me/mediapr/national-survey-of-christian-women-and-body-image/.

[3] Cameron Russell, "Looks Aren't Everything. Believe Me, I'm a Model," *Tedx Midatlantic,* October 2012, https://www.ted.com/talks/cameron_russell_looks_aren_t_everything_believe_me_i_m_a_model.

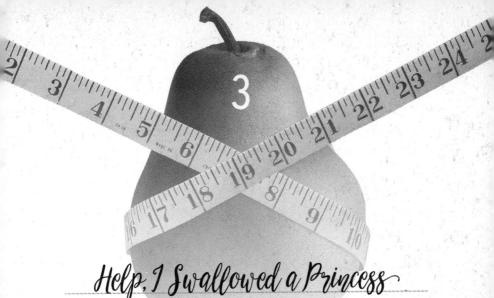

Help, I Swallowed a Princess

"Whatever comes," she said, "cannot alter one thing. If I am a princess
in rags and tatters, I can be a princess inside. It would be easy to be a
princess if I were dressed in cloth of gold, but it is a great deal more of
a triumph to be one all the time when no one knows it."

—Frances Hodgson Burnett, *A Little Princess*

It may be a little nerdy, but I get giddy over a well-planned event.
This one totally fit the bill.

Cotton-candy-colored tablecloths with delicate white plates
and hot pink napkins first caught my attention. Two large tables
spanned the front of the room filled with Barbie princess dolls, and
a bright sign announced to little girls they should take as many
as they pleased. Gallons upon gallons of blush-toned M&M's and
fuchsia candied mints rose to the brim of giant glass vases and
served as each table's centerpiece. Beautifully frosted pink cupcakes rested on tiered white serving stands, begging us to try a
treat from each level.

Everything about this event screamed little girl's dream. My then four-year-old daughter, Katie, and I were invited to a tea party. Not just any run-of-the-mill, sip-from-little-cups-with-your-pinky-out tea party. It was a Barbie tea party.

The media-only event was designed to excite and inform mommy bloggers like me that a new type of Barbie was on the scene: the Barbie Princess. We enjoyed the best hot tea my daughter has ever had (because it tasted a whole lot like warm apple juice) and sampled each of the sweets. While we were making small talk with those seated around us, the emcee interrupted with an important announcement. The guest of honor, Barbie, was joining our party. I could not wait to see how they were going to make a real woman look like a Barbie doll.

To no one's surprise, they pulled it off. She looked perfect to me. I guessed her to be no older than twenty-two. Her long, blonde locks and ball gown almost convinced me. She looked like the Barbie Princess my daughter had grabbed off the freebie table. Barbie gave a cordial welcome. She taught the girls how to smile and wave and then how to curtsy (an important life skill for this millennium). She also gave some brief instructions on proper table setting and good manners—appreciated by every mom in the room, no doubt.

Before the highly anticipated photo ops and her final curtsy *adieu*, Barbie proclaimed she had something very important to tell the girls. She asked them to listen carefully. Her sage advice: always remember there is a princess inside of every girl.

Ooooh. That's good, I thought. Her words sat for a bit. We clapped and headed home.

An hour later, back at our house, my daughter excitedly dumped her goodie bag. (Calling it a "bag" is a gross understatement, as it was larger than the carry-on I used for my last flight.) She then organized her large pile of dolls, Barbie DVDs, posters, and stationery. I noticed that each carried the same mantra: there is a princess inside of every girl. Since my daughter couldn't read yet, I thought I'd point the statement out to her. *Never too early to make sure she knows she's special, right?*

"Hey sweetheart. Did you see this? Did you hear what Barbie said? There is a princess inside of you!"

With an accompanying facial expression that I didn't understand until she spoke, my little girl emphatically said these words back to me. "Mommy, I didn't eat a princess!" And that's when it hit me. Even after a lesson in literal versus figurative language, perhaps this whole "princess on the inside" concept wasn't the most effective way to communicate to my daughter that she was valuable.

Stumped, I had nothing else profound to say on this subject. Suddenly overwhelmed with the reality that Katie may someday have to fight the same body image battle that I have fought, I realized all I had to offer was the same stale clichés of my culture. I possessed no other brilliant words of help beyond, "Hey, you are a princess inside! Look in there until you find her." Oh, and "No, that doesn't mean you ate Cinderella."

If Not External, Then Internal

Candidly, I thought Barbie's princess inside mantra was weak. I offered it to my daughter because I had nothing in my arsenal to replace it. I don't think I'm alone.

The broader truth is, I bought into most of popular culture's methods of addressing the body image problem. Part of me believed the answer to all of our comparison and body image problems was hidden in changing the object of my comparison. If somehow I could see that *she* doesn't look perfect, then I would no longer stress about *me* not looking perfect either.

To help me pep up, celebrities and pop culture leaders offered what seemed like encouraging support. I bought it. In fact, most of the women I know, even those in church, subscribed to these answers culture offered, too. Cameron Diaz got on TV and told me that once I discovered that my cells need carrots more than cookies, I'd find new healing.[1] (Sorry, that fact was not mind-blowing enough to solve this girl's body challenges.)

Others said just write a list. Write which of your body parts you like and focus on those.

It was an okay list.

My feet. (*Well, sort of, but only when my toenails are painted.*)

My smile. (*I've heard I have a nice smile.*)

My teeth. (*The top ones at least. The bottoms need Invisalign.*)

I added a few more minor parts to the list. But it wasn't enough. The list resembled a bridesmaid's dress I once tried on. I came out of the dressing room feeling like this taffeta purple mermaid gown looked okay on me only to hear the bride say that the dress did not "distract enough attention away from my problem areas."

Fail.

Figuring out what I liked about my appearance did not make me forget all that I didn't like.

The *Today Show* spent weeks convincing me (and their millions of viewers) to "Love Your Selfie." I just needed to get happy with the real me I saw in pictures. Overanalyzing the size of my arms or squinting and staring at my photos from every angle to see if my chin was taking over more territory is so last decade. Now, double chins are hot. You love "whatever you got."

Sorry, inspirational morning show crew. That didn't work either.

Everyone's advice-mobile seemed to drive me to the same destination. I needed to love and admire myself more. Then, upon arriving in love-myself-land, I should remember that it didn't really matter what I looked like on the outside because true beauty was on the inside.

What? Which is it? Do I convince myself that I'm hot, or do I convince myself that being hot doesn't matter?

I watched the television show segment on loving me—just as I am. But then they'd cut to commercials that shouted Cover Girl would make me flawless, Weight Watchers would give me my "life" back, and Special K could help me look good in a bikini. (This, incidentally, would help me find an amazing amount of happiness at the beach. I'm quite convinced the woman in that bikini has never attempted to take four children to the beach. I digress.) I read the magazine article on how my personality and spirit are what make me truly beautiful, but then flipped the page to see an airbrushed model showing me how to look great in this spring's styles, followed by a list promising "Ten Ways to Have a Better Body."

All these mixed messages confused me.

My heart is like a memory-foam mattress. Self-love pep talks would make an impression, but then quickly it would go back to its original form. I could hype myself up and feel great for a solid day or two. Then I'd grow weary and end up right back at the same place of struggle where I started.

If body image was a disease, I figured maybe I just had a stubborn case of it.

Or, I just had a load of . . .

Self-Esteem Problems

Dr. Jim Taylor, an internationally recognized authority on the psychology of parenting, wrote a piece for the *Huffington Post* in which he gave his perspective on how America has gone self-esteem crazy over the past forty years. Dr. Taylor says we started getting off track in the 1970s when parents latched onto—but poorly executed—the self-esteem concept. Taylor explains that instead of filling children with true self-esteem, our nation had created a generation of kids who look like they have high self-esteem, yet likely do not.[2]

In other words, the self-esteem proved shallow. All children were given first place for participating so no one would feel bad. Yet, along with no one feeling bad, it turns out that no one truly felt good, either. No one was rewarded justly for a job well-done.

According to Taylor, those same experts told parents that they could build their children's self-esteem by telling them how smart, and talented, and beautiful, and incredible they were. ("You're the best, Johnny!") Unfortunately, life has a way of providing a reality check, and children learned the hard way that they weren't as fabulous as their parents told them they were. The result: lower self-esteem and children who were self-centered and spoiled.[3]

His points seem valid. We water down the value of praise in a way that makes me think of a line from *The Incredibles* movie. When Helen tells her son, the young superhero Dash, that everyone is special, Dash sadly replies, "Which is another way of saying no one is."

Special, unique, extraordinary, beautiful . . .

All of these words formerly defined the ways we stand apart. Now, everyone qualifies.

It makes sense. Generalizing that we are *all* exceptional in *every* arena is disingenuous. I'm not fooled and neither are children.

For example, I lack the ability to make art without a computer. I can't draw a decent stick figure. Art class consistently tarnished my otherwise straight A's report card. If I had received awards for my lousy art—even as an eight- or nine-year-old—I would have known they were meaningless. As a byproduct of accepting an undeserved honor, I may have also questioned my value in other areas. "I know drawing is not my gift, and yet, I won this prize. Does this mean that my other awards were undeserved, too?"

In our culture's kindhearted efforts to prevent anyone from ever feeling like a failure, we may keep anyone from ever genuinely feeling good. We get tangled up in the "nice" trap. We want to be "nice" to everyone so no one loses the soccer game and no one goes home without a prize. But in so doing, we diminish the ways our Creator made us different. We lose our uniqueness. And, likewise, I fear the self-esteem movement hinders our ability to clearly distinguish the root of our body image issues.

I Think I Can, I Think I Can

In the seventh grade, a caring English teacher pushed me on to a new path. Mrs. Miller thought I would be great at speech competitions. This may not seem odd now, given my schedule full of public speaking engagements. But the thirteen-year-old Heather was incredibly shy. Just one year earlier, my sixth grade teacher regularly scolded me for not speaking loudly enough when called on in class. Outgoing, confident, or any other adjective you would use to describe someone who should compete in public speaking did not characterize me.

Yet Mrs. Miller knew I could do it. She believed in me. My parents agreed. So I thought I'd try it. Whether in class or at competition, every time I prepared for my turn at delivering a dramatic monologue, I would sit in my chair and chant the following to myself: *You can do it. You can do it. You can win this. You can do it. Come on. Energy. Energy. You can do it!*

Like the Little Engine That Could, I repeated, "I think I can, I think I can," the whole way up the hill. The judges called my name. I sprang from my seat and delivered a robust performance. I got so full of me I exploded. It worked, short-term. As long as the crowds weren't too large or the competition too fierce, I could handle it. But the heart of my personal pep talk sessions was self-edification. I would pray sometimes, but then still rely on my own strength.

Self-esteem's message roots itself in this philosophy. Focus on yourself, love yourself, praise yourself, pat yourself on the back until you believe how wonderful you truly are. Self-esteem preaches we have goodness within. Embrace yourself just as you are, and don't be ashamed of anything. You be you, no matter what. Do what you want. Be who you want to be. You are what's important. You. You. You.

Sounds a bit like humanism to me. Christianity preaches others before self—not a universe with me at the center, but one with God at the center. It makes me wonder if what we've been taught about self-esteem all these years is even biblical.

Self-Esteem: High or Low, Which Way Should the Christian Go?

To best explore the concept of self-esteem, let's first define the terms correctly. Esteem in its active form means to respect and admire. As a noun, it means respect or admiration.[4] It follows, then, that self-esteem would be the respect and admiration of ourselves!

My three-year-old son refuses to be fully potty-trained. So I'm still changing his dirty diapers. To distract him from squirming (which makes that project *so* much messier), I quiz him. "Who loves you?"

He likes this game and the chance to list the name of every family member. He usually says, "Mommy" first, then progresses through every name he can say. His siblings dote on him with affection, so he confidently repeats their names, in varying order, until I stop my questioning. But I keep pressing. I try to get him to say "Jesus," because I want him to know, at the ready, that Jesus loves him even more than Mommy, Daddy, Grandma, and Nana combined.

So I ask him again, "Drew, who loves you? Who else loves little Drew?"

His answer today confirmed that we are all born with a great amount of esteem for ourselves. His response wasn't the name of our Savior. Instead, he said, "Me. I love me." Case in point, made by my (obviously brilliant) three-year-old. Do we really need more self-esteem?

The Bible remains silent on the topic of us esteeming us. In Matthew 22, Jesus says we should love the Lord with all of our heart and soul and love our neighbor as ourselves. No follow-up verse tells us to love ourselves. God's Word assumes we already look out for our own self-interest. It's presumed that we answer the question "Who loves me?" with the answer "Me!"

If a certain amount of self-esteem is required for healthy living, the Bible fails to spell it out. I regularly hear some Christians talk about the need for increased self-esteem, yet, on another day, I hear other Christians discuss the necessity of decreasing self-esteem. Should it be high? Should it be low? The whole concept seems a bit confusing.

Look at high self-esteem, for example. We can all name someone who qualifies for this status. I don't know about you, but I prefer to avoid the person who thinks (and acts like) she is truly something special. Conversations always focus on her favorite subject—herself. "Enough about me. Now, let's talk about what you think about me!" isn't far from the truth with these people. Love spending time with them, don't we?

Or you may read this and think, "Good thing I don't have that problem. My self-esteem is low, not high. No way could I be confused for the obnoxious God's-gift-to-mankind person described here." But low self-esteem bears more likeness to arrogance than we care to admit. One author explained it well when he pinpointed that the person with low self-esteem actually has the same problem as the person with high self-esteem. She spends too much time thinking about herself and feeling like she deserves more. Though it doesn't seem like the one with low self-esteem has a pride problem, she actually may.[5]

Our first year of marriage confirmed this difficult truth for me.

Making a lifetime commitment to love and serve another person highlights our own level of self-focus in a *special* way. Never before was it so obvious how much I preferred to love and look out for myself first and above all others. In fact, marriage functions as a magic decoder for what hides in our hearts. We are loaded with self-interest that we are able to keep hidden until we put on those wedding rings. Then our partner starts rubbing us (read: annoying us) in a way that exposes our secret.

My pride, selfishness, and fear were uncomfortably revealed during those first few months (and years—yes, it took years) of legal couple status. I realized just how much I cared about things like always being right, getting in the last word, and winning. Low self-esteem, high self-esteem—either way, it seems like a journey that leads us to a destination the Bible prefers us to avoid—self-focus.

Self-esteem sounds healthy, but it masks pride. And when I see Christ-followers embracing the popular ideals of self-love, I'm saddened. We can't expect to find freedom from our body-image bondage by becoming more prideful. Pride is never God's solution to any problem, including our body image woes.

The best example of this happens a few times every year when a woman without a "bikini body" (according to culture's standards, at least) will make a viral showing on social media by wearing her two-piece with pride. The #LoveYourBody hashtags start flying on Facebook, and even my Christian friends tweet how proud they are of this woman for loving herself enough to wear what she wants to the beach. It *seems* like we should applaud her because she's not overly worried about her appearance. That sounds Christian, right? She must be on our team. *Someone press like on that photo, quick.*

But we miss the distinction. The opposite of body hatred isn't body love. They are two sides of the same pride problem. If we want to experience true body freedom, having more body pride will never be the way out. Spending more time esteeming ourselves cannot be the best answer.

Is Self-Esteem a Hoax?

I hope to convince you that, for a Christian, self-esteem isn't the solution. But, just in case conventional wisdom still tempts you, let me show you some proof that self-esteem doesn't work.

What if I told you that although more young people report body image struggles, this same group actually reports higher and higher rates of self-esteem? While a Cornell study shows that 90 percent of normal-weight college-age women are dissatisfied with their body and wish they were thinner,[6] the number of college students with high self-esteem is on the rise. One annual study compares self-esteem of US college freshmen to freshmen in years past. It found that students today are more convinced of their own greatness—regardless of their actual accomplishments. They *assume* they are above average.[7]

For more than thirty years, the myth of self-esteem's value has circulated without data to back it up. Perhaps you even had to take a self-esteem class in school. If you lived in California and grew up in the 1980s, then you may well have. During that decade, the state spent hundreds of thousands of dollars on self-esteem training in schools, believing the investment would make a difference in the state's crime, substance abuse, and teen pregnancy rates. The theory was, once people feel good about themselves, they won't hurt each other, use drugs, or engage in risky, early sexual activity.

Only problem? It didn't work. What happened instead was that the program had virtually no impact on California's social ills. One reporter who followed the state's journey stated the following:

> There is precious little evidence that self-esteem is the cause of our social ills. . . . Those social scientists looked

hard . . . but they could detect virtually no cause-and-
effect link between self-esteem and problematic behavior
whether it's teen pregnancy, drug abuse, or child abuse.[8]

In other words, boosting self-esteem didn't reduce California's social problems.

Still, low self-esteem gets the blame for many of our culture's problems. Every time I Google "body image problems," I can't help but read some multi-degreed person's assessment that low self-esteem leads to eating disorders, suicide, and addictions. Our culture generally accepts that within the concept of self-esteem rests both the disease and the cure. It's the common vernacular. Yet, there seems to be no push to match this rhetoric with the research. The self-esteem movement has made no obvious attempts to adjust their position.

Even *Psychology Today* attempted to discredit self-esteem as the answer to all of society's woes. In a 2008 article called "Self Esteem Doesn't Make Better People of Us," a psychotherapist cites several astounding studies that further disprove self-esteem as our answer. He goes so far as to quote other experts who affirm that no other generation (referring to those born in 1980 or later) has been born with a higher sense of self-esteem, and how this may ultimately be more destructive than good. Over-inflated views of oneself and one's value leads to misery. A 2005 study published in *Psychology Today* demonstrates that it may actually be high self-esteem that leads to societal ills, not low.[9]

Author Jay Adams makes this observation for Christians concerned about self-esteem: "While there is no concern evidenced in the Bible about people having too little self-esteem, and therefore no directions for enhancing self-esteem, God does indicate that He wants us to evaluate ourselves—so far as it is possible to do so—accurately (Rom. 12:3)."[10]

Let's Stop Building Self-Esteem

I love Jell-O, especially all the red flavors. The opportunity to eat Kool-Aid with a spoon? Now, that's a real treat. I have friends (one I married), who can't handle the texture of Jell-O. But its plasma-like consistency fascinates me. *Oh, and it tastes good, too!*

Putting your anchor in the gospel of self-esteem is like filling your mouth with a large spoonful of Jell-O. In the mold, the Jell-O appears solid, colorful, and appealing. But, even with a mouth chock-full of the sweet dessert, there's nothing to really bite into. It squishes around and then mysteriously dissolves. As Dr. Taylor astutely noted in the quote included earlier in this chapter, the self-esteem we offer our children (and personally chase) lacks depth. It has no meat and no roots. It's a house without a foundation. Like Jell-O, there is nothing to sink your teeth into.

I've decided that building self-esteem isn't the right answer for me or for my family. I believe preaching self-esteem to our kiddos just sets them up for disaster. Picture children as balloons. We blow compliments and shallow encouragements into them until they get all filled up with the air from our stale breaths. The balloon grows bigger, just like a child does, but it also grows more fragile. Just the slightest prick of resistance and all of that air disappears. The balloon pops, and there's nothing left.

Let's compare that to what it's like when we esteem our Savior—when we show our children that Jesus is the only one worth praising. Then, we fill them with a solid understanding of the gospel, humility, and God's great worth—not our own. To me, this resembles filling the balloon with water—call it living water, maybe. Although still somewhat fragile (let's face it: people are frail), a water balloon is a whole lot harder to pop. You can throw it. It can bump up against things that are prickly, but it can withstand some adversity. It has a thicker skin. And, when it does burst, something good actually comes out of it.

Jesus is the only lasting treasure. Esteeming anything else or anyone else doesn't offer a permanent solution.

Princess Propaganda

On the surface, the princess movement makes a lot of sense. Our society's battle with body image has damaging repercussions we can't ignore. So telling our daughters that they are princesses on the inside seems like a way to combat the body image issue internally versus externally.

I guess I should like it—a lot. *But, I don't.*

The whole princess movement seems so coordinated in its efforts that I wonder if it was master-planned. It's a ridiculous scenario to imagine, but picture Disney, Mattel (Barbie's family of origin), and even some folks from the evangelical community getting together for a secret meeting to find a common solution. The conversation could have gone something like this.

Disney big shot: "Hey, people are saying that girls are bullying each other and struggling with insecurity. Is there something we could sell them that would make us obscene amounts of money—er, help solve the problem?"

Barbie's people: "I think you were making progress with Snow White and Cinderella. Maybe we just need more princesses?"

Random representative of the evangelical church assigned to attend this bizarre meeting: "Princess? That's awesome. That totally works for us. We have a verse or two for that. Love it."

Disney big shot: "This is going to be big!"

This collaboration obviously never happened, yet somehow all these entities still succeeded in getting our daughters to embrace princesses. It's worked well. Really well, in fact. New cartoon princesses are introduced regularly and yield billions in sales from merchandise alone, just for Disney. I can only assume that

Barbie's version and the Bible verse-inscribed princess tiaras lining Christian bookstore shelves also made nice sales.

It's just not working for anything other than sales. Though moms like me think we help our daughters by filling them with all things princess, in reality it's ineffective. Data shows that during the past thirty years of Disney, Barbie, and even churches pushing "You are a princess" propaganda on little girls, our issues have only compounded.[11] Somewhere between the ages of six and ten, our daughters stop smiling and twirling in front of the mirror and start questioning whether or not what they see is good enough. Feeling insecure about their bodies, our daughters resort to early sexual activity, sexting, bullying, cutting, drug and alcohol abuse, and other destructive behaviors and habits to find affirmation and fill that emptiness inside.

The royal label we plaster all over our daughters doesn't stick all the way through adulthood. I've witnessed, firsthand, a room full of self-focused, modern, would-be princesses.

Will the Real Princess Please Stand Up!

Travel back with me to the Barbie pinked-out room I described earlier. Amidst all of the pretty decorations and delicious treats sat a host of little girls with their hair perfectly coiffed and their frilly designer dresses occupying more of the seat than their tiny bottoms.

They knew how to smile politely. They knew how to stick out their pinky fingers when sipping tea. To the common passerby, the room appeared to be full of royalty-in-training.

Looks can be deceiving.

When it came time to line up, girls pushed and shoved each other to get to the front. When they announced, "Come get your goodie bag!" I had to rescue my terrified four-year-old from getting trampled by older girls who had no consideration for anyone they mauled on their way toward the prizes.

What's even harder to acknowledge were the thoughts that swirled in my own heart at the time. I would like to say that, had my daughter been bigger, I would have encouraged her to politely allow others to go first in that gift bag line. But, in truth, I cared a whole lot about us getting our fair share. Come on, free stuff? We women know the way it goes. "First come, first served." And, "Get yours before they are gone!" These are the accepted rules of the bargain-hunting elite.

No one has to encourage me to think of myself before others. It's in there, deep.

I helped my daughter look like a princess. But not act like one. The concept of princess I asked her to embrace behaved like a toddler-in-a-tiara. This type of princess revels in her own reflection and thinks of herself before anyone else. She is spoiled, self-centered, and entitled. Even if she did like herself, chances are no one else would. (Narcissists make for horrible friends and spouses.)

My friend, this is where we miss it. Being a princess isn't about our posture, pretty clothes, or outward beauty. Not at all. The actual title of princess is bequeathed upon a young woman for one of two reasons. Either she was born into royalty as the daughter of the king, or she married a prince. In either case, her royal value is not intrinsic. She's a princess only because of her relationship with the king.

Picture for a moment Princess Kate, the Duchess of Cambridge. Serving the sovereign Queen of England is her royal duty. She attends diplomatic events on behalf of the monarchy as they ask and instruct her to do. Although she is physically beautiful and by all accounts a wonderful lady, she cannot base her princess status on her grace, looks, or fashion sense. Instead, her proximity to the throne gives her royal status.

The Bible tells us that God sees us as his children (2 Cor. 6:18). But the princess concept, biblically speaking, is the same. The daughter of the king must find her esteem in him, not in herself. His position bestows on her great worth. Proverbs 25:6 (niv) states, "Do not exalt yourself in the king's presence." This amazing truth has great potential to start a princess movement that could actually be effective. And not just for our daughters. Maybe for us, too.

Think with me about a time in your life when you felt really important. Maybe your boss chose you for a special project or a day when someone special in your life did something meaningful. Maybe you received an award or honor for one of your talents. I remember the first time I was invited for a meeting at the White House. My meeting wasn't with the president or even the first lady. It was with a staff person—one about my age and pay grade. But I felt special by virtue of the fact that my name made the list, and I got "cleared" to enter at the back gate I'd seen in episodes of political dramas like 24.

Just being *associated* with a White House staff person for the purpose of *one* meeting was enough to make me feel significant and smile big. I wonder what my posture would be like if I went to the White House all of the time and actually met with the president. Or, better yet, how confident would I feel if the leader of our nation was more than a business associate? What if he was my father?

Sometimes I fail to remember that I'm the daughter of the king—not just a head of state—but the actual King of Kings, Creator of the universe. More so, though, I forget the important One in that equation is not me. I can feel confident because of my connection to the throne, just as I felt important because of my one-day White House clearance. But my value isn't inherent. Even as a princess, my worth still comes from my relationship with the king.

He Is Important

When I think about all the foolish ways I've tried to enliven myself or my children by placing value in our human importance instead of esteeming the incomparable value of our God and Savior, I'm reminded of one of the most famous quotes from the movie *The Help*.

One of the lead characters, Aibileen, works for a family with a young daughter, Mae, who is frequently scolded by her mother. Aibileen nurtures Mae and calms her tears by reciting the following three sentences with her, "You is kind. You is smart. You is important." It's a beautiful interaction in the movie. We are supposed to be touched by the way Aibileen does a better job of pouring into Mae than her own self-centered mother. It's very effective. After watching, I resolved to come up with my own equivalent of those three sentences for my daughter.

Yet, as God continues to work on my heart and reveal to me the cure to my worldly struggles—including my regular fight with my physical appearance—I see that the answer isn't found in how "I is." Rather, it is who *he* is.

Chapter Mirror

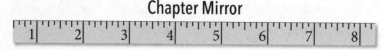

Many cite self-esteem as the problem behind body image battles. But increasing self-esteem, from both a biblical and effectual standpoint, fails to solve our body image issues. Both high self-esteem and low self-esteem lead us to the wrong destination in our body image battle: a place of pride. Meanwhile, culture and the church have used the concept of "princess" as a way to reinforce the message of self-esteem and help girls grow confident. The message falls flat and reinforces the ineffective message of self-esteem to our daughters. If we want to see true freedom from our body image struggles, we need to forsake esteeming ourselves and pursue esteeming the king.

Heart Exercises

This week we are going to examine what the Bible says about self-esteem and self-love.

1. Before reading this chapter, did you think of self-esteem as an unbiblical concept? Why or why not?

2. Read 2 Timothy 3. What does this chapter say about self-love? What does it associate self-love with?

3. How often do you feel you've been told that you have to love yourself or think about yourself first? Do you see this instruction as biblical or out of step with God's commands? What other examples of the self-love movement have you seen in our culture?

4. Read Romans 8. Make a list of how life in the Spirit differs from life in the flesh. How do you think this applies to messages of self-esteem?

———————————————— ～ ————————————————

Memory Verse: "Do nothing from selfish ambition or conceit, but in humility count others more significant than yourselves" (Phil. 2:3).

Notes

[1] Cameron Diaz, "A Healthier You on the Inside and Out," *Today*, February 26, 2014, http://www.today.com/news/healthier-you-inside-out-cameron-diaz-positive-body-image-2D12164199.

[2] Jim Taylor, "America's Self-Esteem Problem," *Huffington Post*, June 10, 2010, http://www.huffingtonpost.com/dr-jim-taylor/americas-self-esteem-prob_b_607718.html.

[3] Ibid.

[4] "Esteem," m-w.com, retrieved April 2014, www.merriam-webster.com/dictionary/esteem.

[5] Edward T. Welch, *When People Are Big and God Is Small: Overcoming Peer Pressure, Codependency, and the Fear of Man* (Phillipsburg, NJ: P & R Publishing, 1997), 32.

[6] Cornell University, "Most College Students Wish They Were Thinner, Study Shows," *ScienceDaily*, accessed March 2, 2017, www.sciencedaily.com/releases/2007/11/071120111544.htm.

[7] "How College Students Think They Are More Special Than EVER," *Daily Mail*, January 5, 2013, http://www.dailymail.co.uk/news/article-2257715/Study-shows-college-students-think-theyre-special--read-write-barely-study.html.

[8] David L. Kirk, "Lack of Self Esteem Is Not the Root of All Ills," *Santa Barbara News-Press*, January 15, 1990.

[9] Michael Formica, "Self-Esteem Doesn't Make Better People of Us," *Psychology Today*, May 17, 2008, https://www.psychologytoday.com/blog/enlightened-living/200805/self-esteem-doesnt-make-better-people-us.

[10] Jay Adams, *The Biblical View of Self-Esteem, Self-Love, and Self-Image* (Eugene, OR: Harvest House, 1986), 113.

[11] Eating Disorders Coalition, "Facts about Eating Disorders: What the Research Shows," Eating Disorders Coalition (website), accessed May 22, 2015, http://eatingdisorderscoalition.org.s208556.gridserver.com/couch/uploads/file/fact-sheet_2016.pdf.

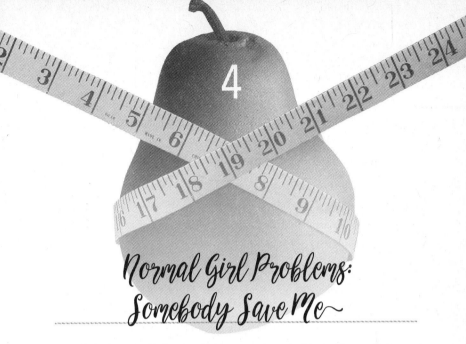

Normal Girl Problems: Somebody Save Me~

"If I find in myself a desire which no experience in this world can satisfy, the most probable explanation is that I was made for another world."

—C. S. Lewis, *Mere Christianity*

To celebrate our eighth wedding anniversary, my husband and I spent the night at one of the coolest hotels in Dallas—the Omni. I love fancy hotels, and this one—with its magically appearing television in the bathroom mirror and under-the-nightstand lighting that only flicks on the moment you step out of bed—suited me just fine.

The next morning, we ventured over to another Dallas hotspot called Klyde Warren Park. The perfectly manicured green space sprawls a few city blocks and nestles among the tall city buildings. Food trucks line one of its perimeter streets, as do dozens of tables with chairs. By one of the children's playground areas sits an outdoor library, where you can pick up a book or magazine to read while you enjoy the park's serenity.

Though I had brought my own reading material, it seemed more fun to first browse the library's offerings. The latest issue of *Time* magazine captured me with its cover photo. I tend to lose track of current events. Maybe I should catch up, I mused. I grabbed it and sat down beside my already-reading husband. The sun illuminated our table and felt hot for early October. I rolled up the sleeves to my T-shirt—to prevent farmer's tan—and continued flipping through the pages.

A few minutes later, a group of women filling the table next to ours distracted me. People-watching interests me *so* much more than *Time* magazine. One woman pushed the coolest metal stroller I'd ever seen, while another motioned at older children to stay on the closest side of the playground. A third came alone. She chirped a few "hellos," then apologized for wearing her workout gear. She had come straight from the gym. They settled in with small talk, and I went back to looking at my magazine. After all, it's not polite to stare.

Current events. Blah, blah, blah.

Then their conversation turned interesting. (Well, at least more interesting than the article on campaign finance reform. Yawn.) I didn't stare, but I sure did scoot my chair a few inches closer to their table while leaning their direction to hear better. When one of the women said, "If I could only lose this baby weight!" my antenna went up. Reading morphed into a guise for my eavesdropping. (Uh, I mean my "book research.")

"I just hate the way my body looks since I had her!" the woman with the trendy stroller lamented. She looked stylish and trim to me, wearing cute patterned capri leggings and a long solid-colored tee.

Her friend, the one sporting workout gear, said, "Oh, you still look great. I haven't even had a baby, and you're still thinner than I am."

New mom had no reply to that. So the third woman chimed in, obviously a mediator. Though she seemed to only half-listen while watching her older children play, she attempted to talk some sense into both ladies. "It's harder once you have children. That's for sure. But I think we all struggle with liking the way our bodies look. There's nothing wrong with either of you. You both look great. These are just normal girl problems. All women struggle. We always will. It's just the way we are."

Normal girl problems?

All women struggle?

It's just the way we are?

Hmmm . . .

That's what I used to think, too.

A Typical Story

When people would say, "What's your story?" I squirmed. *Awkward.* What do you say to that? I didn't know if they wanted me to talk about where I went to school or past jobs. Or maybe they expected me to tell them about my upbringing or the different cities I called home. It always seemed like a vague question for which I didn't really have a great answer.

I felt very normal. Average. Not extraordinary.

Christian people asked me for a different kind of story: my testimony. Frankly, I felt lost once again. Raised in a believing home, I told my mom I wanted to say the sinner's prayer together before I could dress myself. I'd heard enough "real" testimonies to know mine didn't qualify. It included no stories of the wild life I survived pre-Jesus. No list of addictions from which he saved me would captivate an audience. I frequently began my answer with the disclaimer, "Well, it's not really that great a testimony. See . . ."

I envied people with phenomenal conversion stories. My Marine husband surrendered his life to Christ in a tent on a military base in the Middle East during Operation Enduring Freedom. He could clearly point out what life was like before and after Jesus entered the scene. Others could testify to the ways he changed, too. But my story always made me self-conscious. I know others have far more dramatic plot lines, characters, and themes.

Now I feel differently about it. The journey God has taken me on to find a way out of my body image issues has become a part of my story. Although my rescue may not capture Hollywood's attention, to write it off as less necessary would be to proclaim my own self-righteousness. I needed a Savior as desperately as the addict, just as urgently as the prostitute, and just as despairingly as the dying. Freedom eluded me until I recognized the severity of this need.

This is my story.

My Normal Girl Problems

I stood in front of the full-length mirror that occupied the corner of my bedroom and stared at my thighs. I remember, quite vividly, the scene. I always felt big, even though I actually wasn't. My thighs were mostly to blame—my thighs and the pants. The pink pleather pants I wore to my third grade class that day only made the problem more obvious. I loved those very stylish pants (it was the 1980s). Yet I hated those pants because I felt like my bottom half looked too conspicuous in them. Oh, and they were hot—extremely hot. (If you've never experienced so-called "vegan" leather pants, they seriously don't breathe. At all.)

When I picture middle school me, I visualize a girl much chunkier than the one I see in my seventh or eighth grade class picture. My face was too full, my eyes were too small, and my bangs were too flat. (I did mention it was the 80s, right?) It only takes a few minutes of staring at the photos before my mind goes back to the same thoughts it had when I first viewed the class photos more than twenty years ago.

I could summarize my high school experience as vanilla. I never talked to anyone about my struggles with my body. I just did what I knew to do and tried to be a good girl. I played sports and enrolled in just about every extracurricular activity offered at my Christian high school. I made excellent grades. A firstborn rule-keeper, I never did anything too wild that would get me into real trouble.

I became more aware of my weight during high school and experimented with food to control it. I'd overeat in the evenings and then wake up feel guilty and resolve not to eat the next day. Buzzing through the morning without eating was no problem. Then I occupied myself at noon so I just didn't have "time" to eat during our lunch period. I'd return home and binge, ruining all of my efforts to starve myself. Since in my estimation I had already blown it, I'd eat dinner as normal. (Plus, this habit kept my parents from ever noticing anything too unusual.)

In addition to my oversized thighs, my chest was too small and my nose was too short, not to mention square. Combine all of this with my weight and a mole on my wrist—the size of a pencil's eraser top—and you have a comprehensive list of the obstacles I thought I needed to overcome to find happiness in my life at age sixteen. I wish that some part of that last statement was exaggerated—any part of it, really. I'd diet, pinch my nose to make it thinner, always wear black on the bottom, and buy the most stuffed push-up bra around to try to have a fighting chance. On special occasions, I either put concealer over that mole or would wear a bracelet that would stay in place over it. I searched for the mole in photos and got upset if I, somehow, forgot to put my left hand in just the right spot to cover it.

College for me started just two weeks after I turned seventeen. Not wanting to worry about my weight while there, I got as thin as I could before school started. Yet a small body didn't help me overcome my insecurity. Overwhelmed and lonely, as most young college students are, I could only figure out one way to help that lost feeling—eat! Food comforted me, and college life afforded me many opportunities to stay by its side. Everywhere I turned I found an opportunity to eat. With a cafeteria full of prepaid options and a dorm room full of junk 24/7, I easily put on the freshman fifteen and then some.

I packed on twenty pounds during that first semester. This started a cycle of gaining weight while I was away and then coming home during school breaks to try to lose it. The cycle took its toll on my body. I went most of my sophomore year without getting my period. A normal reaction would be, "Hey, there was something wrong. Why didn't you get help?" But in the nineties, eating disorders were only for the very thin or those who binged and purged. I didn't fit either description.

Diet pills weren't as taboo during that decade, either. In my senior year of college, I started taking a supplement to help increase my metabolism. I exercised occasionally, and the pills gave me more energy to get through workouts. The night before fall break, I took some of my new metabolism boosters and went to the gym. Zipping with boundless energy, I was able to do two strenuous aerobics classes in a row without tiring. When I returned home, I couldn't sit still. I couldn't focus. I couldn't think. I aimlessly wandered from room to room throughout my small campus apartment. I couldn't keep my attention on one thing long enough to finish it, like eating dinner, dressing for bed, or sorting through the giant pile of clothes (that week's reject outfits) that covered my desk. I needed to pack for a weekend trip, but focusing on what I should take for just a few days away proved impossible. Feeling out of control and scared, I remorsefully (because I liked the way they helped me lose weight) stopped taking those pills.

The fullness of my face and figure tarnished my graduation photos. What they revealed embarrassed me. With my degree now finished, changing my body would need to rise to priority status. My life as a yo-yo dieter continued even though school breaks no longer helped me focus on weight loss.

My first job title out of college read: deputy press secretary. I worked for a US Congressman on Capitol Hill in Washington, DC. For a few weeks, I felt important. I lived in the mix of the biggest power brokers in the country. I ran into (literally, I mean the walking-right-out-of-the-elevator-and-finding-myself-face-planted-into-some-important-guy's-tie kind of run into!) men whose names and faces you would immediately know.

But as the weeks turned to months, I realized that entry-level work, even in an exciting place, stifles a creative spirit. Spending all day long in front of the copy machine discouraged me. I turned to food to get by. The restaurants in the office buildings offered a great selection of comfort foods, including dirt-cheap frozen yogurt, the perfect accompaniment to my sixty-four-ounce Diet Coke each afternoon.

Slowly my diet and sedentary lifestyle, combined with a bad habit of feeding my misery all evening, led to a packing on of pounds. Fortunately, I was so well-versed in dieting that I always had a new program to start—on Monday, of course. (Unless it's January first, everyone knows there is no better day to start a diet.)

On the rare occasion I could move from my post in front of the copier, I sat at my tiny desk and stared over at our office kitchen. I made mental lists of new food rules to follow:

I will no longer eat the donuts they bring on Monday
    mornings.
I will no longer participate in office pizza Friday.
I will drink only water. Hmmm . . . (I couldn't live without
    Diet Coke.)
Change that. I will drink more water.

Each time I foolishly hoped that my new weight-loss quest would be my last. I desperately longed for the permanent solution so I could just be thin and happy forever. Happiness came from being skinny. As did love. I knew the only thing standing between me and my dream of finding true love was that disdainful number on the scale.

I thought about my weight all of the time. A constant conversation played in my head, reciting how much I weighed and what I needed to do to lose it. I felt guilt as I calculated my calories for the day or pride as I congratulated myself for only eating half the pint of Ben & Jerry's. My brain focused on food, the scale's digital readout from that morning, and my "fat" body during every lull of the day. All other goals, hopes, and dreams for my life paled in comparison to my dream of being thin or, as I really meant it, being beautiful. In fact, from the age of eighteen to thirty-one, the first resolution on my list every New Year's Eve was to lose weight.

And comparison, it consumed me. Everywhere I looked there was someone thinner, prettier, or more successful than me. I spent most of my free time shopping for "magic" clothing that would help me look thinner so I could feel better about my body. If I wasn't out shopping, I was consuming the latest *Self* or *Shape* magazine to read what foods I should avoid to make myself more beautiful.

Aerobics Instructors Aren't Insecure

Exercise and I shared an interesting relationship. I knew it helped me lose weight and feel better. But I didn't think I was good at it.

I felt clumsy and uncoordinated. I run like a duck, with a terribly short stride. I once threw up after a 5K race. (I wish that said marathon. But, no. I may well be the only person in history to have ever overexerted herself running three miles at a terribly slow pace.)

My monthly income working on Capitol Hill amounted to around ten dollars more than I needed to pay the rent alone (which meant sharing a house with four other women). The local gyms knew the crowd—poor Hill staffers like me—so they offered a bargain membership with one catch. You could only work out after 9 p.m.

No problem. I could do that. The gym sat only seventy-five steps from my townhouse's front door in the city's southeast quadrant. So I ran there and back every night. (Scared to be out alone, after dark, I somehow thought my *lame-o* running would keep me safe.) Within a few months, exercise became a new savior. Working out afforded me something no diet could—the freedom to eat all I wanted (including my daily frozen yogurt) and not have to buy new pants every two weeks.

When you idolize something like fitness, you realize there are people who serve as priests in your new religion—the personal trainers and aerobics instructors. Though not in great shape, I made it a personal goal to someday become a fitness instructor. The concept of getting paid to work out seemed sort of genius. I reasoned that once I attained that level in my exercise walk of faith, then I would never need to diet again. Becoming an exercise professional meant freedom from the weight and body image struggles that plagued me. If my name tag read "Aerobics Instructor," then I would finally be saved.

At age twenty-eight, I passed the (surprisingly difficult) written test to become a certified group fitness instructor. I started teaching Spinning and kickboxing classes at age twenty-nine. I had arrived. Unfortunately, it didn't feel as good as I assumed it would. In fact, standing up front and leading classes while sporting a headset microphone didn't really satisfy me. I still compared myself to women in my classes who were more fit. I still didn't believe I was thin enough.

If Only Prince Charming Would Come and Fix This

I spent the remainder of my twenties bouncing from job to job and moving from place to place across the country.

The pace of Washington, DC, wore me out, so I sought a break from fifty-hour workweeks in graduate school. But I tired of schoolwork and sitting in class after only a year. Restless and anxious to get back to the crazy pace of politics, I packed up everything I owned and drove to Abilene, Texas, to run a US Congressional race. As soon as the votes were counted, I moved back to DC to see if fulfillment would come for me the second time around. It didn't. So, after another year passed, I headed west again to manage another US Congressional primary in Oklahoma.

When I returned to DC for the third time, I felt more discouraged and confused than ever. My career had already experienced its share of ups and downs—big jobs and good salaries but crushing losses. Political work is not for the faint of heart. I managed to keep my weight under control through a combination of diet and exercise. (Revolutionary. *I know.*) Though I'd be lying if I said I didn't think about it a whole lot. The biggest discouragement—what haunted me as I committed to yet another job in the nation's capital—was that age thirty loomed on the horizon, and I still wasn't married. This felt like rejection, and it slowly destroyed the paradigm I built for myself. My formula promised that if I stayed thin, then I would get married and have a family. I couldn't figure out why it wasn't working.

Instead, my life followed a different track, namely, career building. My master's degree, vast work experience, and resume meant little to me. I wanted a husband. I longed for rescue. A man would surely save me from my loneliness. I craved someone who could answer the deeper cries of my heart. Those questions it asked like: Am I beautiful? Am I valuable? Will anyone ever love me? I naively thought a man could answer these in such a way that I'd never have to ask them again. (Ten years into marriage, saying that is laugh-out-loud funny.)

God didn't answer the send-me-a-husband prayers I prayed from age seventeen to thirty-one. But, shortly after my thirtieth birthday—the day I feared would confirm my eternal singleness—God allowed me to meet him.

A successful Marine fighter pilot, a workout zealot, and a smart guy who loved God—I won the love lottery. Our easy courtship led to wedding planning after just eight months. I taught a lot of side aerobics classes, in addition to my full-time job, to help pay for my dream wedding. Combine this with my newfound ability to sustain myself on love rather than food, and I, like many brides, was in the best shape of my life on my big day.

But we married and something very strange happened. I tangibly felt it the morning after our wedding night. I woke up and glanced at the clock in our ornately decorated hotel room. I noticed my new husband still lying there beside me. Palpably, something was missing. From the bed, I could see myself in a small mirror above the vanity. My glamorous hair and make-up from the day before were destroyed. My dress, now piled up in the corner, was filthy from taking photos outside. Instead of feeling fulfilled, complete, and whole—finally—I just felt like the same old me. The person staring back at me in the mirror wasn't any different. The contentment marriage promised certainly hadn't arrived on day one.

Nor did it arrive on day two or day twenty or day one hundred. In fact, I soon found that getting married hadn't cured all (or any) of my insecurities. Within twenty-four hours of saying our vows, I wondered if I was too fat for my new husband. Though his behavior did nothing to legitimize my fears, my brain worried over thoughts of whether or not he actually liked my body and whether he was somehow disappointed in me already.

Marriage, a husband, these were supposed to be my secrets to body image freedom—the end of my physical appearance worries. Once my wedding band slid onto my left hand, I obsessed even more. I realized I had competition, other women—everywhere—who were prettier and thinner. He would see them. He would know the truth. What if he wanted better? How could I know if I was enough?

Comparison corroded my soul and just about ruined my brand-new marriage. I took my insecurities out on him. I insisted he do better at making me feel valued. I griped and whined. I guilted and browbeat him into doing more to prove his love. I couldn't handle any criticism. I couldn't handle any hint of disagreement. (Yet I frequently picked fights.) I constantly worried that he would leave me and, in some ways, I thought maybe I could speed up the inevitable.

You could aptly describe me as a crazy, self-absorbed new wife who was blessed with a patient husband. Desperate for affirmation, I pressured him to answer those questions of my heart. Yet he couldn't do it to my satisfaction. He was unable to convince me of my value or worth. He could not prove his love or my acceptance in a way that offered me permanent assurance.

Marriage was an investment portfolio where I put every last dollar of my hope. I planned for my husband to yield great dividends for my empty soul's account. Yet he couldn't deliver.

You Won't Care about Weight When Pregnant

What does every insecure new bride need to do? Get pregnant, of course! Our four-month anniversary barely passed before I decided to pee on a stick and confirm what my bloated and achy body insinuated.

I always wanted to be a mom. But still jilted by the way my expectations of marriage let me down, I was nervous to pursue any additional dreams lest they also shatter. Terrified describes more accurately how I felt when I read the word "pregnant." Add some hormones to that fear, and the mix made for an angry, emotional, impossible-to-please-for-the-whole-first-trimester type of pregnant woman.

Yet another myth I believed for so long was soon to be classified as fiction. Certainly pregnant women didn't wrestle with body image. Once I was with child, I would never worry about my body size and shape again. Right? Moms occupy a different category—or so assumed my pre-pregnant self. Why would a woman with a husband and children be overly consumed with her appearance? I knew most were not. How could they be? (Four children later, I find this, too, ridiculously funny. In fact, a recent study showed that moms are actually more concerned about their body image than the rest of the population.[1] It only took me two trimesters of pregnancy to confirm this data through personal experience.)

I gained mass faster than a bowl of frozen yogurt at the pay-by-the-ounce place. I felt out of control in the weight arena for the first time in years. I didn't like it. Though eating for two (or twelve is probably more accurately how my calorie counts would divide) seemed liberating, I obsessed over every pound revealed on the doctor's office scale. The number that arrow pointed to disturbed me so much that I scheduled my office visits for the time of day when I knew my weight would be lowest. I got aggravated when the nurse rounded the number up instead of patiently waiting until the scale balanced in between the two digits.

I had a problem.

I added fifty pounds during my first pregnancy. It felt awful and sucked the joy out of having a baby on board. I had no appreciation for the blessing who was on his way. Worry about my weight consumed me. I'd see pregnant women on the cover of magazines and compare my bloated and obviously pregnant-all-over body to their petite frames and cute baby bumps.

My next child started incubating just months after my first arrived and the cycle continued. Over the course of the next six years, I spent all but a handful of months either pregnant or breast-feeding. Controlling your weight when pregnancy and nursing hormones run your body is like trying to diet while on an all-inclusive vacation—difficult.

During this time, I also first began fighting for and finding freedom. I considered myself a Christian. Raised in the church, I was taught that "It's what's on the inside that counts." I just had no idea how messed up my insides really were. I knew how to fix my body but had no clue how to fix my heart. If I did (indirectly) confess my insecurity or body image struggles to another Christian, after telling me that my true beauty was inside, he or she would also say things like, "Just pray about it!"

So, I prayed: "God, help me be thinner."

"God, please help me stay on this diet and really lose the weight this time."

"God, please help me to be more disciplined and exercise more." Yes, I prayed a lot.

"God, why can't I just be one of those 'naturally' thin people who don't need to worry about this kind of thing?" And what I normally meant was, "God, it's not fair that you gave me this body I hate! Why didn't you make me beautiful?"

"God, can you send me a man to fix this mess I feel inside?" I had begged him a thousand times. I meant a husband, of course.

But later I realized I got it wrong when the one whose name I took couldn't make my insecurity disappear.

Now I understand God's perfect response to my request. I wanted him to send a man to save me from my struggles.

And he always responded, "I already have."

The Gospel Surprised Me

I thought I knew the gospel. I certainly could have recited it for you backward and forward. But I had no idea how to apply it to my life. In many ways, I was a Pharisee. I knew the law, so I tried to live as morally as I could. I paid a lot of attention to my actions. I paid very little attention to my heart.

I didn't realize how my body image issues kept me bound and, truthfully, dead. I couldn't experience the freedom of new life in Christ because I was held captive to the belief my answer was in fixing my appearance. I tried to justify myself by making my outside pretty enough to earn acceptance. It's been my experience that a lot of self-named "good girls" like me never ventured into obvious rebellion, yet still engage in a desperate search for worth, value, and joy in ways contrary to God's plan. I'm not proud of my distorted thinking or the desperate ways I searched for fulfillment. If you read this and face a similar struggle, know that the answer and real hope await you.

Maybe your struggle looks different. Perhaps God already revealed to you his glory and your own depravity, yet you wrestle to figure out how your body image battle relates to the other struggles he's saved you from. Let me encourage you that there's hope for even greater freedom.

I acted Christian-like but not Christlike. My relationship with Jesus was ambiguous and hollow. I knew how to listen to the Holy Spirit and let him guide me, but I missed the meaning of grace. I easily understood justice. But getting what you don't deserve?

Incomprehensible! Reticent to like it, I didn't really believe I needed it. After all, I was "good." My journey to comprehend salvation—and freedom—started in biblical counseling. Looking back, that's the only place the hardness of my own heart could have been touched. Admitting I qualified as a sinner—not just a forgive-me-for-sneaking-a-cookie kind of sinner, but someone who needed rescue—helped me get started.

What I believed about myself was wrong. I thought I needed my appearance, a husband, or a family to save me. I thought the number on the scale or my fitness credentials would give me the joy I desired. Frustration perpetually ensued as these idols let me down. Freedom came only when I realized that my struggle rested in my heart. I didn't want a Savior. I wanted salvation to come on my terms, in a way that I could control.

In church, I said things like, "God, you have my everything." Or, "Lord, I'll do whatever you ask." But I could never surrender my struggles with body image. I could never figure out how he would fill that void and answer my questions of worth and value. I needed to be taught how the gospel applied to my life so I could be free. Like Elsa in the movie *Frozen*, I needed to learn how to "Let It Go."

Eventually, God brought me to a place where I realized his plan of salvation for me included redeeming me from the bondage of body hatred and the trap of comparison. He showed me that Jesus died for my sins and that among those sins were my so-called "normal girl problems" that included not liking my shape and compulsively exercising, dieting, and obsessing over how to change it. I finally realized the joy he had in mind for me *far surpassed* the happiness of fitting into a single-digit size.

I believe he can do that for you, too.

Chapter Mirror

Salvation brings us freedom, but in Heather's story, we see she didn't find freedom because she was looking for it in all the wrong places. God desires to set us free even from the mundane, "normal girl problems" that plague us. He is the only place where we'll find true salvation.

Heart Exercises

Read Acts 13:38–39 and Romans 3:21–24.

1. Are there areas in your life where you're in bondage? Are there specific struggles that weigh you down, consume your thoughts or time? List them here.

2. How do you define the term freedom? What do you think that would look like in your life?

3. Do you believe you can find freedom in your areas of struggle? Why or why not?

4. Take some time this week and pray about this question, "Does my heart derive its worth and value from Jesus alone?" If you struggle to say yes, consider and write down the reasons you hesitate to find this answer.

———————————————— ∼ ————————————————

Memory Verse: "I will walk about in freedom, for I have sought out your precepts" (Ps. 119:45).

Notes

[1]Melissa Dahl, "Stop Obsessing: Women Spend Two Weeks a Year on Their Appearance, TODAY Survey Shows," *Today.com*, February 24, 2014, www.today.com/news/stop-obsessing-women-spend-2-weeks-year-their-appearance-today-2D12104866.

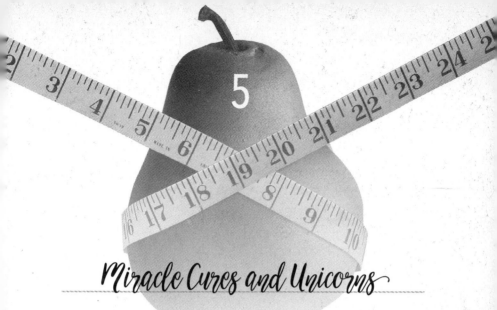

5

Miracle Cures and Unicorns

"We have a right to believe whatever we want,
but not everything we believe is right."

—RAVI ZACHARIAS

Charlie didn't have a chance at finding a golden ticket. Only five of them existed—hidden in chocolate bar wrappers—and four had already been claimed. Even if he had that kind of luck, his family didn't have money to buy frivolous treats like candy. If Charlie were anything other than a character in a classic fantasy movie, I'd tell him to get real and give up the dream, dude.

But if you've seen the 1971 version of *Willy Wonka and the Chocolate Factory*, you know that Grandpa Joe *does* find a way to get a Wonka Bar. In spite of great anticipation, the packaging doesn't contain one of the coveted golden tickets. Then something amazing happens. Charlie finds a discarded Wonka Bar wrapper. Inside, he discovers the final golden ticket. This leads the duo of grandfather and grandson on a bizarre, life-altering journey where strange things happen to greedy children.

Of course a movie about a chocolate factory would move me. But what on earth does Charlie's adventure have to do with you and me and body image woes? It's like this: I'm always searching for golden tickets. Not literally, of course. Though if someone could invent a weight-loss product that tasted exactly like Dove chocolate, I would buy stock in the company and then hoard as much as my attic would hold.

Opportunistic? Perhaps.

Sometimes I surprise myself with my own lapses of naiveté. As fitness professional for over a decade, my desk holds a pile of paper certificates that claim I am well-versed on topics like exercise, diet, and weight management. Yet when I see a headline that touts, "Lose 15 pounds in 4 days!" I'm intrigued. I wonder if maybe *this* one could actually work. I wonder if *this* formula will be *my* golden ticket.

I watch an infomercial that tells me an exercise gizmo will give me rock-hard abs in just five minutes a day. (*That's right, just five minutes a day*!) I have to physically restrain myself from grabbing my credit card to make the first of four easy payments of $19.95.

The bottle of diet pills boasting, "Eat what you want and lose weight" in a giant yellow font screams at me from the store shelf. I grab it, hold it in my hand, and even spin it to find the price before I talk myself back to reality.

What's my problem? My brain knows these quick fixes are nothing but folly. But my heart wants them to be true. It longs to believe two false premises.

First: My heart wants to imagine that somewhere out there a golden ticket does exist—an easy way or "miracle cure" that will forever free me from my struggles.

Second: It wants to believe that *true* freedom *is* freedom from my earthly struggles—that simply having the right number on the scale brings joy, and happiness comes from wearing a size four.

My heart resembles the child who still believes in Santa. She tidies up to make room around the fireplace and sets out cookies, milk, and a sweet note. My heart desperately wants to believe in magic because it longs for more than this life has to offer. Can you identify with this struggle? This longing for more? If so, you can understand my tendency to grasp for even the craziest of Ponzi schemes.

Or, as I like to put it: I chase unicorns.

Not the pretty, one-horned equine that flies. No, my unicorns are the fictitious ideas that stir my *desire* but are not based in reality. My erroneous, magical thinking quickly and easily turns into my heart's idols.

> If I were rich . . . then I'd be happy.
> If I were thin . . . then I'd be happy.
> If I had this type of car . . . then I'd be happy.
> If I had a husband . . . then I'd be happy.
> If I had a baby . . . then I'd be happy.
> If I had a baby who slept through the night . . .
>   then I'd be happy.
> If I had two babies and a bigger house . . .
>   then I'd be happy.
> If I had a husband who would help me take care of these
>   two babies and our big house . . .
>   then I'd be happy.

Please, tell me I'm not the only one who has felt this way.

Stop and think about what your heart believes would make you "truly" happy. If you have a quick answer that's anything other than Jesus, then you too may be chasing unicorns of idolatry.

Our idols tempt us. They lure us in by telling us they have incredible experiences in store for us, if we can just make it a little further down their path. If we can just lose a little more weight, make those abs a little firmer, get those boobs a little fuller—then they'll deliver. But once we reach the milestone, they respond with, "Good job getting this far, but it's not quite enough. Keep trying! I'm sure you're almost there."

They dangle the prize of all that we truly desire—like contentment, acceptance, and peace—in front of us until we've travelled so far from the place where we started that we no longer recognize who and where we used to be.

Idols lie. Whether they are idols of body image, life, children, marriage, your home, your finances, they all continually lie. And, for women, the idol of beauty seems to plague us more than the others. If you idolize beauty or if you think you need more beauty, I hope you'll keep reading. In this chapter, we will grab a big shovel to dig out and expose what's really at the root of our body image and comparison struggles.

First: Understand That Beauty Isn't Bad

Humans have an innate love for beauty. God put deep within our hearts the ability to discern and recognize it. After all, he formed all of creation. He gives us beautiful things, and he makes all things beautiful. Have you ever noticed how we have the ability to discern beauty even in things that don't meet society's definition of beauty? Let me share an example.

For years I was a loyal *American Idol* fan. Some nights I even voted—multiple times! (Don't tell anyone. I'm sure forty-year-olds are not supposed to be that committed to reality television contestants.) During a recent season, the gorgeous singer, dancer, and actress Jennifer Lopez served as a member of the judge's panel. Though Jenny from the Block obviously feels a need to prove herself in the "sex symbol" arena, as a judge she offers humor, encouragement, and grace in her critiques of even the worst of the singers.

Even if you've caught one season in the past fifteen years, you know that the *American Idol* powers that be seek much more than just the next amazing voice. They want someone with the whole package. Usually this equates to someone who can transform into a glamorous entertainer with the right clothes, hair, and makeup.

In the past few weeks, I watched Jennifer tell two different contestants they were beautiful. This surprised me because, by Hollywood's standards, neither of these two performers seemed to come close to measuring up. One, a young African-American man, carried eighty pounds or more of extra weight. Right after she told him he was beautiful, she made the most fascinating remark. "You grew up in the church, didn't you, baby?"

The guy smiled politely. "Yes, ma'am."

"I could tell. I can just see that light."

I gasped when she said it. As much as we try to fault Hollywood for forcing an unattainable standard of beauty on us, one fact remains. We know true beauty when we see it. J-Lo knew only to call it light. (Which technically was right.) How many times have you seen that same light shine through a child with a severe handicap or in a woman from a different culture who has no knowledge of our fashion or makeup trends, but in whose eyes and smile you see true beauty?

In some ways, beauty is completely subjective. Just like the old adage proclaims, "Beauty is in the eye of the beholder." Yet, in other ways, we know when we experience the real thing. We respond from a deeper place when we encounter beauty of a different level. In Psalm 27:4 David talks about "gazing upon the beauty of the Lord." Although a cultural standard of beauty often distracts us, we can recognize a heavenly standard of beauty.

The same principle holds true when you observe a physically beautiful person acting in a degrading or distasteful way. Miley

Cyrus serves as one example, but the list of women blessed with great physical beauty who can use it in an ugly way grows annually.

Our spirits sense true beauty. Yet, we need to guard against a subtle shift that can take place as we observe it. We can easily cross over from the side of appreciating or recognizing beauty to the worship of beauty—which is neither healthy nor holy. I don't mean lust, although it certainly qualifies as a way our heart can stumble into sin. Rather, for many who struggle with body image, I think we've fallen into the trap of misplacing value. We worship beauty instead of the Creator who makes all things beautiful.

Second: Find the Heart of the Matter

Please don't misunderstand me. I'm not against beauty or beauty rituals. I don't think God gets mad when we dress up for a special date night or get a facial.

The Bible does instruct women not to make their beauty come from their outward adornment (1 Pet. 3:3). Yet we misinterpret this Scripture when we read into it that we should look sloppy and unkempt. You can (and should) be a good steward of the body God has given you. Instead, this verse teaches against an overemphasis on outward appearance. It's the type of chastisement Jesus gave the Pharisees who counted on their public actions (long prayers and lots of religious-sounding talk) to justify them before God. His warning: our physical appearance can't save us. Nor will it, ultimately, score us lasting points with our husbands (or future husbands). Only a gentle and quiet spirit achieves that (as the passage continues to clarify).

Peter also wants to emphasize that if we spend all our time in the gym, nail salon, and Macy's—to the exclusion of reading our Bible, spending time in fellowship with other believers, and praying and communing with our Savior—we may try to *look* beautiful, but we miss the mark.

Have you ever met a woman you thought was really gorgeous until she opened her mouth? Or, to the contrary, have you ever met a woman who at first glance you thought was a little plain, but then once you got to know her a bit, her spirit made her quite attractive? Peter wants us to remember this. Physical beauty doesn't *ultimately* make a woman beautiful.

So where does our struggle lie? It comes down to what we value. In the Bible, the term is *treasure* (Matt. 6:21) and Jesus tells us that where our treasure is, there our hearts will be also. Is Jesus upset if we have a drawer full of cosmetics and a couple of shape wear items? I don't think so. Rather, his desire is that we don't become so encumbered in beauty that it becomes our heart's pursuit. He wants our hearts free from other entanglements to pursue him alone

So, let me ask you. Where is your treasure?

Putting a disproportionate amount of our resources, effort, and time into the beauty quest signifies misplaced treasure. Instead of Jesus, beauty becomes the treasure we seek. Our hearts get off-track. Culture likes to use the term *balance*. But this concept can deceive us. Balancing the time or money you spend on beauty to the amount of time or money you spend on entertainment may be one way to tell where your treasure is, but it's not the best activity to put on the other side of the scales. What if you weigh the time you spend getting ready every morning to the time you spend connecting with your Savior through Bible reading or prayer each morning? (That's a tougher test, one I'd fail most mornings!)

Even good things can become bad things when used incorrectly. I think about one of the Bible's most famous verses on money. Some interpret it to mean that money is bad, but that's not what the verse says. It reads "the love of money is the root of all kinds of evil" (1 Tim. 6:10). The same applies to our physical appearance. Loving (prioritizing, cherishing, chasing) beauty above all else causes the harm. Ranking our physical appearance over spiritual growth sets us on a destructive path. Our cosmetics bag doesn't determine whether or not we have crossed the line over to beauty worship—our hearts do.

Third: Recognize What Hasn't Worked

We were twenty-five and single, so we decided to go on a cruise, just because we could.

My dear friend Heidi and I were going to enjoy seven days and nights lying on Caribbean beaches, eating delicious dining room food, exercising in the ship's gym, and enjoying the services of a world-class spa. During our first day at sea, I pranced into the spa to make an appointment for a facial. A few minutes later, I walked out of that spa with appointments for not only a facial, but also for a funky water massage and a revolutionary new anti-cellulite treatment that would take inches off my thighs in just one hour. (Yes, I realize that sounds hokey. But, trust me, those spa employees held PhDs in persuasion.)

A few days later, I donned the fluffy white spa robe and slippers, then journeyed back to a room that sounded and smelled like it was in the middle of a rainforest. My technician came in, turned down the volume on the thunderstorm soundtrack, and pulled out her measuring tape. *Yikes. Was I paying for this humiliation?* She started by taking measurements of my thighs, my arms, and my stomach. She planned to target these areas with the special seaweed potion, she explained. She assured me the measurements were important so that I could see the great results at the end.

Well, this seems promising. Surely they wouldn't go to the trouble of using a tape measure if it didn't work! Right? This must be legit.

Soon the sounds and smells in the room changed as my hour of an anything-but-relaxing treatment began. I can't remember it all, but it included a vibrating belt thing, heat, slimy seaweed, something else that smelled like it came from the ocean's floor (and not in a good way) that would extract toxins out of my skin to make it tighter. My esthetician pushed and pressed and rubbed and pulled on me. Then she cleaned off the seaweed for the moment of truth.

What would the measurements reveal? She grabbed the tape measure out of her white jacket pocket.

Success!

I had somehow lost an inch off each thigh, a half-inch off my upper arms, and two inches off my stomach.

Wow! That is phenomenal. Where do I leave my tip?

I returned to my cabin smiling. Heidi asked if I thought it worked. I felt my thighs as I looked at them in the cabin's full-length mirror. *Did my shorts actually feel a little looser? Maybe?* I remained optimistic.

"Yes, I think it did."

The more I scrutinized my body, the better I felt about my results. My confidence soared as I pulled on my black cocktail dress. We walked down the ship's corridor toward the dining room, and I patted my thighs every few minutes, still energized by their new firmness.

Heidi and I sat down at our assigned table with the same couple we had dined with for the past few evenings. We chit-chatted about tomorrow's shore excursions and the features on the menu. And then it happened. The very thin and attractive woman sitting across from me smiled big and said she had a great day at the spa because she had tried a phenomenal new spa treatment.

Uh oh.

With some hesitation, I asked the question. I feared the answer, but I could see she wanted to share her results. Fairly confident her outcomes couldn't compare to mine, I invited it. This woman didn't have a spare inch to lose from anywhere. It was safe.

"So, how much did they say you lost?"

With giddy exuberance, she reported that her results were exactly twice as fantastic as mine. For every inch I reported gone, she lost two!

I deflated faster than an unplugged bounce house. Not because her results were better, but because this woman was Q-tip skinny. Her results were not possible! I had to face the fact that I had fallen for a hoax.

A gimmick.

A rather expensive gimmick, actually. *But you probably already knew that.*

Miracle cures are so very tempting. I feel confident sharing my naiveté in falling for the seaweed-lose-inches-in-an-hour scheme because I know you may have been fooled in a similar way. Our desperation for results leads us to do some silly things—some rather expensive silly things.

You've likely heard the hackneyed definition of insanity: doing the same thing over and over again and expecting different results. Every time I hear this saying, I think of my tendency to chase unicorns. I spent my teens and twenties searching for the cure like a song set on repeat, sure the next diet would yield lasting results. The next fitness program would work for life. I needed every latest exercise gizmo. (Yes, I actually owned a Thigh Master, a Total Gym, and an Ab Roller. I also made my fair share of "easy" payments for a slew of other workout DVD programs.) I devoured hardback diet books.

Yet it didn't work. The cycle never ended. Instead, I found a newer way to lose weight and a newer food I should or shouldn't eat. An improved exercise plan would beat out the old one (that I had just finished paying off). So desperate for a miracle cure, I forgot that none of it ever lasted.

I needed a new way out.

Don't Tell My Heart, My Achy Breaky Heart

I became a country music fan living in Washington, DC. (I know. It's odd that the city brought out my country side.) But the Texan friends I was surrounded by taught me something they referred to as two-stepping. (Although I've done it dozens of times, I'm still not sure what those two steps are . . . I digress). About this time, a country star named Billy Ray Cyrus (who would later be referred to only as Miley's dad) released a song called "Achy Breaky Heart." It's kind of a silly song if you haven't heard it, but it has a whole choreographed line dance that goes with it. The country dance places would play it between the slower songs.

Through the lyrics, the singer tells his soon-to-be ex-girlfriend that she can tell everyone they are finished, just don't tell his heart. His heart wouldn't understand, something the song explains in a countrified way. I find it amazing how aware we are that we can lie to ourselves, but we so often want to leave our hearts out of it. In fact, we spend a lot of time defending our hearts and trying to persuade ourselves (and others) of their goodness.

No one likes to blame the emotional and soul-filled part of her heart for anything. How romantic it seems to talk about following our hearts wherever they lead, or simply trusting our hearts. We foolishly assume that our hearts will always take us down the right path. While "Listen to Your Heart" makes for a catchy pop song chorus, it's just not biblical. Jeremiah 17:9 says the heart is deceitful and desperately wicked and asks, "Who can understand it?" The psalmist suggests we "guard" our hearts. James 1:26 tells us we can deceive our own hearts into thinking we are religious. We can't trust our hearts, nor can we follow them. They're to be watched as closely as a three-year-old around an open package of Oreos.

I've followed my heart down some pretty shameful roads. I wanted some things so badly I deceived myself with the idea that God was making a special exception to his rules for my short-term happiness. He wasn't. God doesn't bend his laws for us. My heart lied. Your heart does, too. Like a smooth-talking Italian waiter working for tips, it tells you all kinds of things that will lead you into trouble if you believe them.

We can't win body image battles through a hostile takedown of all external pressures that nip at our heels. Nor can we achieve lasting victory by (finally) finding the right diet or the "guaranteed results" exercise plan. We fight the real battle, the ground war over our body image, in our hearts.

The Secret Combination

My daughter Katie owns a pink metal safe for all her seven-year-old-girl valuables. Covered with script font-printed stickers that say "top secret" and "no boys allowed," it has a combination lock to provide *maximum* security.

It's not a modern push-button lock, but an old-school one, with a circular knob and an intimidating clicking sound. You must stop precisely on the right numbers in sequence to make it work. You know you got it right if you hear the loud unlatching noise, followed by an irritating ring at the final stop. The worst part? She can't open it or even remember the combination. Fortunately, it's printed on a sticker on the bottom. (I don't know how those Barbie clothes, Polly Pocket dolls, and plastic bead bracelets can possibly feel safe with protection this careless.)

These locks make me a nervous mess. Trying to open it, I'm transported back to high school and my red gym locker that would never cooperate. I panicked after a few failed attempts. If it wouldn't unlatch before the bell rang, I faced a fate almost worse than death—I'd have to wear my gym clothes for the rest of the day! My problem: I prefer estimation to the exactness required by combination locks. Turning it left and stopping directly on the unmarked line that is sixteen, and then turning it just a few notches back to six. That's way too much pressure.

Over the years, as I heard women talk about what they had to do to "get over" their body image issues, I treated this news as if they were divulging a secret combination. I listened attentively, writing down every word.

Three clicks left of "Love your body."

One full spin of "Embrace your curves."

Two clicks right of "Be kind to yourself."

Spin it left back to "Accept who you are," then take a half-turn counterclockwise while saying, "God made me beautiful."

Whatever their formulas consisted of, they never worked for me. Desperate, I tried all of them. *At least twice.* But I felt like Dorothy clicking my heels and chanting, "There's no place like home." I'd follow the directions, open my eyes, and discover I hadn't been magically transported anywhere.

I needed to get that method just right because I desperately longed for freedom. I consumed every book I could find. I listened to every speaker. I smiled at myself in the mirror. I got in touch with reality by studying the airbrushing process. I read the statistics on what size, shape, and weight characterize the average American woman. I stopped criticizing pictures of myself. (*Okay, out loud at least.*) I took everyone's advice and did everything that *anyone* suggested I do. But nothing worked. Disheartened, I fought depression each time I realized that another new method would also fail.

For this reason, I hesitate to offer a one-size-fits-all solution for our body image struggles. God meets us where we are. Words that bring inspiration and healing to one woman's soul may fall short at helping another woman's struggle. I also don't want to pretend to give away a secret combination, because there isn't one—at least not a secret one. I refuse to bill this as a miracle cure. But, at the same time, I *know* that if you follow the steps prescribed here, you will find yourself on the path to freedom because the Bible guarantees it. God's promises are better than any money-back guarantee.

The solution I present to you here—and throughout the remainder of this book—follows a pattern laid out by Scripture on how we handle the issues in our lives that keep us in bondage. The answer comes straight from the Bible. If you've been in church for a while, you may already know these passages. Yet I think it will surprise you. In my decades of searching, this solution was never on any list. That's just one reason I'm excited for you to try it!

The Elephant in the Room

This is the one gigantic elephant in the room that will help a great number of women . . . if they will only acknowledge it. No one wants to be the one to risk saying it. I get it. In fact, in previous chapters I've danced around it. I may have mentioned it in passing. This job isn't fun. I'd much rather tell you something "encouraging." I'd probably sell more books that way. But I'm going to give it to you straight. Are you ready for this?

We have to confront the roots of our body image issues as sin. We have to call them that, and then repent. Do you want to be free from this struggle? Then address the sin. Name it, repent, and get on the road to freedom.

Ouch! Are you surprised? Please follow me here so you can clearly see it, too.

Ephesians 6:12 says that we don't wrestle with flesh and blood but that our battles are spiritual. I don't believe our battle to be beautiful is different than any other kind of sin struggle.

It's not a battle of us versus them—the women who struggle with their size versus the underwear models. Not at all. (That's just another reason comparison hurts us in the long run!) Our body image battles are an extension of the epic battle in our hearts of good versus evil. The propensity of our hearts to chase and desire beauty is just as much a struggle against our sin nature as the tendency toward greed (desiring more money) or substance abuse (desiring comfort from a thing other than God).

When our hearts are lured toward desiring anything other than Jesus, the Bible uses two words. One is *idolatry*, which we'll discuss at length in this chapter. The other word that you've likely heard more in the context of body image is *vanity*. A derivative of that word—vain—often classifies a woman who spends a lot of time worrying about her appearance. But the Bible's definition of vanity is broader than just a woman who looks in the mirror a lot. It encompasses everything we pursue that won't last beyond this earth.

Look at James 1:11, where the author talks about meaningless pursuits withering like the grass under a scorching sun. All of our struggles with our weight, our nose shape, our leg size, or whatever it is about our physical bodies that we think would bring us contentment if we could magically change them, are simply vain pursuits, fruits of our flesh. Could it be that our battle to be beautiful, our mental wrestling matches with insecurity because of the way we look, are all just ploys of the destroyer of our soul designed to keep us from pursuing Jesus and his will for our lives?

Idolatry 101: Something Make Me Happy, Quick!

You probably aren't surprised that chasing beauty is a vain pursuit. But you may still be wondering where the actual sin is in your longings to be thinner, prettier, or curvier in the right places. Ready for this? It's called idolatry. And if you are totally lost on this whole idolatry concept, don't worry. I was, too.

Dr. Timothy Keller, the pastor of Redeemer Presbyterian Church in New York City, has written and preached a lot on the topic. But until I started listening to his teaching, I hadn't really considered idolatry a relevant topic for this century. Here's how Dr.

Keller defines it: "Sin is building your life and meaning on anything, even a very good thing, more than on God. Whatever we build our life on will drive us and enslave us. Sin is primarily idolatry."[1]

I knew the Ten Commandments, but I convinced myself that the one about idols only applied to Moses's followers and their propensity toward worshipping inanimate objects. Oh, and people in other cultures. I could clearly identify idolatry on the other side of the globe where people bowed to gaudy gold statues or cows. (Cows? Really?)

I had never considered the possibility that *I* could be an idolater. My home was statue-free. I didn't even have a garden gnome. Just to be safe, I averted my eyes as we walked past the Buddha statue at the Hong Kong Express.

Modern-day idolatry erodes our souls without us even realizing it. In fact, once you recognize it, you'll start to see it everywhere—at the mall, at professional sporting events, in people's homes, and at work. God designed us as worshippers because we were created to worship him. But, much like those Israelites in Exodus who decided a golden calf would be fun to bow down to, we bow to other much more "important" things now.

Do you have friends whose toddlers' sports schedules run their lives? Or know a guy who can never miss his team's game? Or have a friend who never says no to anything because helping people is where she finds her identity? Modern-day examples of bowing our lives to people, things, work—everything other than Jesus—are everywhere. We erroneously believe that our idols can bring us life. Why? Because we sense a brief feeling of happiness when we "worship" them. But they can't keep us happy. We long for more, so we push our idols to give more and do more. In vain we long for our idols to satisfy us.

Here's the tricky thing. Most of the time, idols aren't bad things in and of themselves. Like I said before, God created beauty. It's not a bad thing. In fact, idols *can* start out as very good things or even *blessings* from God—like husbands. But, like I shared in my story, I so desperately needed a husband for fulfillment that when I actually found a man to marry, he had no chance of filling that void. He couldn't satisfy me because I put him in a spot he wasn't designed to fill—that of savior.

If you have children, you may also be tempted to make your family your idol. I love my children deeply. I would throw myself in front of a bus or bullet for any of my four blessings. But if I start to derive my value and worth from my position as their mom, then I am crossing the line into idolatry. If my happiness or livelihood depends on them, I'm a family idolater. Feeling worthy of love on days when my children behave well or, conversely, feeling like a failure when a day is filled with rebellious tantrums, could serve as a barometer of my idolatry. My identity can't be rooted in my status as "mom"—it too needs to be rooted in Jesus.

Want to know what you idolize? Ask yourself these questions: What do I treasure? What is it that I absolutely cannot live without?

Do you have a hard time spending money or giving money at church? Maybe you idolize money. If you feel overly connected to an individual person—a parent or friend—maybe you have put them in the wrong place as responsible for giving you "life," and you need to make an adjustment. If you think the scale's readout, a different number inside your jeans, or a new body will give you life, joy, or peace, then you may be a body image idolater. There's a quote by an archbishop named William Temple that says something like this: your religion is what you do with your solitude.

You may want to read that again and let it sink in.

It took a while for me to fully grasp what this meant. But once I did, I realized I had a problem. *A big problem.*

I spent a lot of time thinking about my weight, how I could lose weight, what diet I should start, or what food group I could cut out to lose weight. Though I rarely acknowledged my battles out loud, the constant conversation in my head was about my physical appearance and my desire to change it. My religion centered on body improvement. The scale was my god. My heart led me astray. Like that old hymn sings, "prone to wander, Lord, I feel it." I got off-track. I bought (and fully invested in) the lie that if I could just look different, then my life would be better. Never did I think of this as idolatry.

I knew Jesus *said* he had more for me. I just couldn't see past my idolatry to any other, better way.

Temptation and Idolatry

Today I bought my 243rd new bottle of anti-frizz, hair smoothing, straightening iron serum. And in a few hours, I will need to wash my hair for the second time today because, just like all of the others, this new formula made my hair so greasy it still looks wet. *Nice.* Truth is I don't *really* know how many bottles of miracle hair product I've purchased. I just know that I fall for the promise of frizz-free and hassle-free straightening. *Every time.* (Well, at least every time the bottle costs $7.99 or less. I don't do expensive hair products, which I understand could be part of my problem.)

Our hearts are idol factories. All around us we see the promises of happiness, joy, and a better life, so we bite. We long for the express pass to happiness. We want the miracle cure. We take shortcuts, sign up for "get rich quick" schemes, and use our Keurigs because we want gratification, now!

Satan is our tempter. He knows our hearts are drawn to the easy path. He expects us to keep trying the next new thing that promises "amazing results." The enemy whispers in our ear, "He would love you more if you were thinner." Or, "You would be married by now if you didn't have such a big nose." Instead of refuting him, we believe it and become all the more desperate for a miracle cure. We fall for his other lines, too.

If you were prettier, life would be easier.
Your marriage is hard because of how fat you look.
If you would just lose weight, he'd want you more.
If the swimsuit tag read size two instead of twelve, you'd
*   actually enjoy the beach.*
You would have gotten that job if your skin was clearer.
No one will ever love someone who looks like you.

I know these lines because I've heard them. All of them. "No temptation has overtaken you that is not common to man" (1 Cor. 10:13). When Satan says things like this to us, it doesn't *seem* like temptation. It's not like he's trying to get us to commit adultery or steal jewelry. But realize that his lies *are* still taunting us to sin. The false premises that the enemy feeds us tempt us to make beauty our answer instead of Jesus. He tells us that looking more like that magazine photo solves our earthly woes, so we make beauty the treasure we seek. Satan lures us to find our joy, identity, and value in our physical appearance instead of in Christ. And it gets us into trouble every time.

Sydney, a reader of my blog (ComparedtoWho.me), recently shared with me the following story. Sydney's story exemplifies well how the enemy plants body image lies in our hearts early and then continues to feed them as we age.

I was six years old the first time I thought I was fat. I looked at another little girl, both of us in our little jean shorts, the thought crossed my mind, "My legs don't look like hers." And they didn't. My little muscular legs didn't match the little twigs I saw on my friend. Rather than simply noting a difference, I saw a major flaw. I saw fat. I saw bad. Shame about my body quickly flooded in, and that moment marked the beginning of many years of intense struggle with body image.

Little girls find many occasions for wishing . . . blowing out birthday candles, seeing a shooting star, catching a fallen eyelash on your finger so you can blow it off. My wishes were always the same. Every year. I never had to pause and think about my wish. It was always *I want to be skinny.* It consumed my mind.

I look back at the little girl I see in old pictures and am in awe of just how skewed my perception was. I wasn't big at all. It is heartbreaking and it is scary. I never told anyone how I felt about my body. I assumed they all saw me as huge, too, and I would be even more ashamed.

Through junior high and high school I became consumed with food: counting calories and restricting, skipping meals and lying about it, feeling ravenous and out of control when I hadn't let myself eat for an extended period of time, and exercising as much as possible. I aimed to burn off the exact amount of calories I ate. I would come home from sports practices and run however many miles it took for me to break even. I was terrified I would never be able to live a normal life, not engaged in this constant battle with food. I didn't know how to trust my body.

I lost a substantial amount weight my sophomore year of college and hit the number on the scale that I thought would finally satisfy me. But to my shock, it didn't. It was exciting at first, but I still didn't like how I looked, and I was gripped by fear of gaining the weight back. I finally got what I thought I had always wanted, but I was very sick and in jail in my own mind. It was a vicious cycle with no light at the end of the tunnel. I equated my body with my worth . . . a very dangerous association to make.

My eating struggles and negative body image came and went in waves of intensity through the next few years. I was never hospitalized. I was never deathly ill. But I was being completely robbed—robbed of joy, of fun, of carefree moments. I was robbed of the opportunity to focus on things that truly matter. I was robbed of the chance to be confident and free.

It wasn't until recently God opened my eyes to help me see how much was stolen from me. I couldn't even really see other people because I was so busy looking at myself. I was being robbed of the joy of life. I was being robbed of my purpose. I got tired of being robbed and decided to really let God into this battle with me. And only there I have found freedom.

The Gospel Combination

Our hearts resemble my daughter's pink, sticker-covered safe. We keep a lot of junk locked in there, but often we don't know the combination to freedom. We need the code to redeem what is inside. Much of what we've kept trapped (and even protected as part of our heart's desires) needs to be removed and replaced with something better.

Each of us has a different story. Some have wrestled full-blown eating disorders, hospitalizations, and near-death experiences, each triggered by body image lies that take root and choke out truth and life. For others, the struggle may have begun with an unwanted sexual encounter—abuse, rape, or another's cruel behavior planted seeds of body shame that have felt impossible to remove.

For others, there may not be a trigger event or dramatic story of struggle. Instead, little comments over the years have fed the beauty beast. The voices of disgust echo these comments and spread the negative propaganda like a cancer through your mind. "You'd be happier if you could just be thin," they taunt. "You're worthless if you can't lose weight," they lie.

My friend, I don't want to minimize in any way the uniqueness of each of our struggles. Nor do I want to overlook the damaging effects of a harsh parent, abusive boyfriend, or invasive perpetrator. But I do want to encourage you with some hope. No matter the differences in the how, when, or why behind our body image struggles, our answer is common. It's not a secret formula or a combination that's frustrating to unlock. Instead, it's just a turn toward Jesus—moving to a better understanding of what he did for us and how the gospel can speak to and truly heal our broken body image.

In the remainder of this book, we'll dig into this and the other steps toward freedom. In step two, we'll discuss confession and how we truly find freedom from the grip of beauty and body image idolatry. Step three will discuss comparison. Step four will look at changing our habits, and step five will examine how to create healthy community so we can stay free.

**Note: If you've been diagnosed with an eating disorder or suspect you may have one, please read "A Word to Those Struggling with Eating Disorders" at the end of this book and consider seeking additional counsel.

Chapter Mirror

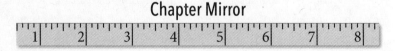

Our natural bent is toward the quick fix, the miracle cure, and the magic solution that will bring us eternal happiness. For many who struggle with body image, we think that cure is somehow related to the way we look. So we chase unicorns, trying to look just right to finally find peace and joy. We do this because our hearts deceive us. The not-so-secret combination to finding freedom may be found in acknowledging our sin of chasing idols, specifically the sin of body image idolatry. Idolatry is when you take something good or bad and make it a thing of ultimate value—something you can't live without. The combination to clearing out the junk of our hearts and finding freedom is found in the gospel.

Heart Exercises

Read James 1 and then answer the following questions.

1. Have you struggled to find the right combination to unlock your body image struggle? What other things have you listened to or tried that didn't help your struggle?

2. Have you ever considered that part of your struggle may be a sin issue? Why or why not? Does the commonality of the struggle make it seem less like a sin issue to you?

3. How would you define modern-day idolatry? In what ways do you think your heart is "prone to wander"?

4. Read James 1:9–11. In the last verse, James talks about our fleeting pursuits. In what ways do you think our body image

struggles are fleeting pursuits that distract us from pursuing our Savior?

5. Spend a few minutes thinking back through your body image struggle. When do you believe it began? Can you identify any trigger events? What lies about your body have you believed? Write out whatever comes to mind here. (Sometimes journaling can lead to greater clarity, so don't be afraid to take your time answering these questions. If you are working in a group, encourage members to read out loud what they've written as they feel comfortable.)

———————————————— ～ ————————————————

Memory Verse: "For the sun rises with its scorching heat and withers the grass; its flower falls, and its beauty perishes. So also will the rich man fade away in the midst of his pursuits" (James 1:11).

Notes

[1]Timothy Keller, *Counterfeit Gods: The Empty Promises of Money, Sex, and Power and the Only Hope That Matters* (New York City: Riverhead Books, 2011), xvi–xvii.

Part Two

The Spiritual Solution

to Body
Image
Issues

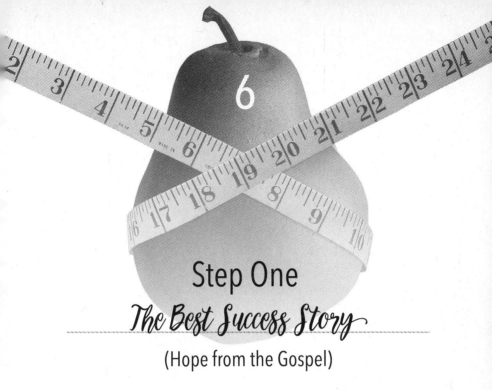

Step One
The Best Success Story
(Hope from the Gospel)

"The disease of self runs through my blood.
It's a cancer fatal to my soul. Every attempt on my behalf
has failed to bring this sickness under control."

—DC Talk, "In the Light"

Do you like a good success story?

I sure do. As a success story addict, I subscribed to two different fitness magazines that featured the encouraging tales and the before and after photos. Every month, I ripped open the surrounding plastic and flipped to those articles. I scrutinized the pictures, noticing every difference, then read what type of diet and exercise combination yielded magazine-worthy results.

Maybe you like them, too. You may have watched television shows like *The Biggest Loser* or *Extreme Makeover: Weight Loss*

Edition—the reality show versions of body transformation. Why do we love success stories so much when, in truth, watching or reading about someone else losing weight doesn't actually help us get any healthier? (Especially not if I sit on the couch watching the show while eating a bowl of cookies 'n cream.) I know *many* people who don't need to lose an ounce of weight, yet they still tune in each week.

Why? Because success stories give us something we crave—hope. They show us that true transformation *is* possible. We desperately want to know that change is attainable, within reach. Success stories show us that miracles *can* happen.

Let's take an even closer look at what these amazing transformations actually offer us. In the context of a weight loss success story, it may look like the plotline is about a man or woman changing his or her life by dramatically changing size. But I think there's more to it than that. I believe these shows demonstrate salvation.

Now, I realize I may have lost some of you there. You are wondering how I went from talking about eating ice cream while watching your favorite weight loss show to heaven and hell in like three sentences. But follow me here. The connection will surprise you.

Take *The Biggest Loser*, for example. If you've never seen the show, participants are portrayed as coming from a background of torment and pain. They struggle with severe obesity and the life hurt and complications that come with it, both physical and emotional. They feel trapped in their own sort of hell. Then their trainers come along—Bob, Jillian, or whomever the hot body helper of the season is—and save these distressed souls from their torment by helping them transform. The show paints a picture of salvation from hell, offered through a savior (their trainer) that leads to the joy, peace, and happiness that accompanies life as a thin person.

Could it be that we read, watch, and enjoy success stories because our hearts also long for salvation?

Watching others transform excited me because I too craved what it seemed like they had found. I desired the freedom, happiness, and joy of the salvation that (apparently) accompanied a thin body. Yet weight loss-anchored salvation couldn't save me. Realistically, a thin body doesn't last for eternity. The freedom it offers is fleeting. My idolatry fooled me into buying this *Biggest Loser* definition of salvation, so I chased it. I thought insecurity would vanish once I wore a size four, got married, had children, or had the rest of my life in order. Then I would feel saved, happy . . . joyful, even. But that wasn't the case. None of these idols satisfied or brought me freedom.

I needed a real Savior.

Sorta Saved?

Granola bars are a bit of a farce. They seem like a healthy snack alternative, but often they are loaded with sugar and they aren't very filling (especially the affordable brands that don't use real nuts and fruit).

My eldest son, Zach, is going through another growth spurt. He comes downstairs an hour after breakfast and takes a bar from the now half-empty, Costco-sized box of chocolate chip bars I bought just last week. I tell him it's too early to start with the granola bars and beg him to eat a banana or have more breakfast instead (since it's only 9 a.m.). But he only wants a granola bar. So, stubbornly, he heads back upstairs empty-handed.

We will repeat this same scenario about eight times today. Each time he'll go for the easy, sugary snack that will leave him hungry an hour later, instead of taking the time to eat something more filling like an apple or a sandwich. If I can catch him in the act, I'll tell him when the next mealtime is ("It's only one hour until dinner, Zach!") and ask him to wait. Then he'll march back up the stairs to ride it out.

Through much of my adult life I hungered for salvation but lived on granola bars. I couldn't understand why my savior wasn't filling me up. So I'd settle for seemingly nutritious snacks every time I felt empty.

Maybe a pedicure would make me feel better.

Maybe this diet pill will lead to joy.

Maybe a shopping trip and scoring some great bargains will fix my depressed mood.

Maybe a facial will help my confidence.

I was too focused on the ways the world promised to save me through improving my appearance. My pride prevented me from admitting that my own sin was keeping me from experiencing the peace my Savior offered.

Ultimately, what I believed about salvation through Jesus was wrong! I knew the gospel backward and forward. Though sinless, Jesus died on the cross to take the punishment for my sins, so that through him I could be justified and put again in right relationship with God the father. *Got it.* But I thought that salvation was, ultimately, for later.[1] The kind of salvation I believed in assured me of where I'd spend eternity, but I didn't think the gospel had anything to offer my present life and my present struggle. Morality oozed from my being. I didn't need to be saved from a drug habit or a corrupt lifestyle. I couldn't see how the gospel had answers for my "normal girl issues" like my quest to look a little better.

No one ever showed me, in a way that I could understand, the connection between Christ dying for me while I was still a sinner and complete acceptance. I never comprehended how Jesus's sacrifice set me free from trying to earn his love (and the love of other people) through looking and acting "good." Now I know that the gospel tells me God wouldn't love me more if I was better (or thinner) and that God doesn't love me any less—even if I'm struggling to obey.

Buried beneath our surface desires to have a better butt, to weigh less, or to tone our thighs hides a longing for something much greater—a desire to feel valuable, to feel accepted, and to feel loved. God put that there. We think that just losing the weight or having plastic surgery will get us the happiness and the joy we long for. But it's never enough. We all need a real Savior to fill our hearts' emptiness.

What in the World Is Worldliness?

I homeschool my children. Not because I think it's the only right way, but because that's what we've decided works best for our family. I thought I'd hate homeschooling. Teaching one hour of children's church on Sunday mornings requires me to hide under the covers for the rest of the day! But I've been surprised how much easier homeschooling has made my life. (Oh, wait, I was supposed to say something about how much better it has been for my children . . . *Yes, that's true, too.*)

During my first year of homeschooling, I figured out how quickly children will tell you what they already know. (Often so they can be finished with their "school day" faster.) I ask them to work on a specific subject, say geography. And my oldest immediately says with groaning for emphasis, "Mom, we know all of that!"

I'm tempted to believe him. But just to be sure, I get out the map. When we start going through each state and its corresponding capital, his tune changes.

"Okay, Mom. We know *most* of our geography," my son concedes.

To find body image freedom, I had to first recant my "expert Christian" status.

Perhaps you are like me and decided to follow Jesus a long time ago. And, like me, maybe you didn't think there was any way that your body image struggles could correlate to all that stuff you learned in church. I was certain my understanding of salvation wasn't the problem. I thought I had it down, until one day, I heard a pastor talk about idolatry in a way I never had before. And then, just like my son recognized he didn't really know his geography as well as he claimed, I realized how the sin of idolatry dominated my life—a sin I didn't even think really existed in my Christian circles. Never before had I seen my heart actively pursuing other gods and actively rejecting the freedom Jesus offered me through his sacrifice on the cross.

I believed that satisfaction would come from a number on a tag, a letter in my bra size, or achieving thigh gap. What Jesus offered seemed good, too, but what beauty offered me held more appeal for right now. That sin kept me separated from God. While salvation was supposed to set me free, I only experienced a small portion of the freedom that went with it. Though my pardon had been granted, I decided to stay and hang out in the cell. Jail offered few luxuries, but at least it was familiar.

In James 4 we are warned against worldliness. I always assumed this had something to do with listening to more Christian music than the so-called "secular." Or not dressing too wild because that would be "worldly." Worldliness was just another reminder for me to be moral. And as a "good girl," this part proved easy. Now I see that this isn't what worldliness is about at all.

The author of James talks about the war within us—the battle between the flesh and the spirit. Let's read James 4:1–4 here:

> What causes quarrels and what causes fights among
> you? Is it not this, that your passions are at war within
> you? You desire and do not have, so you murder. You
> covet and cannot obtain, so you fight and quarrel. You
> do not have, because you do not ask. You ask and do
> not receive, because you ask wrongly, to spend it on
> your passions. You adulterous people! Do you not know

that friendship with the world is enmity with God?
Therefore whoever wishes to be a friend of the world
makes himself an enemy of God.

Let me try to paraphrase this. James isn't talking about wearing longer skirts, listening to more Toby Mac than a rapper named Mac, or reading your Bible for one hour to balance out every hour of television you watch. No.

Instead, he's saying there's a fight going on inside of us. A big fight! And that internal war sometimes makes us crazy. We have a hard time getting along with each other. We compare ourselves to each other and squabble and form cliques that separate us from each other because of this battle in our souls. James tells us why God doesn't always give us what we want—our motives are driven by these worldly passions, not by his will for our lives.

To make this vernacular apply specifically to our body image issues, I'd loosely translate James's words to say something like this: You want to be skinny! You want to be beautiful! But hey! Can't you see how these desires cause strife among you? You ask God to help you stay on your diet or to clear up your skin, but he won't answer because your motives are wrong. You want to change your body to satisfy a worldly desire, not to fulfill God's purpose. Hey, all you who are caught between your desire to look like a *Glamour* cover model and to look like Jesus, choose wisely.

James doesn't tell his readers that it's okay to strive for both— beauty (for the purposes of this book) and God. Instead, in verse 4, he actually calls them adulterers and explains that since they have chosen to be friends with the world they are now enemies of God.

Adultery? Wait . . . surely this good girl couldn't be guilty of that. *Or was I?* Could it be that my affection for beauty and passionate pursuit of a better body placed me in that adulterer category as well?

Mindy's Story

One of my blog contributors named Mindy sent me this message a few weeks after she discovered my blog. Her words capture our battle with worldliness and body image.

> I'm thirty-five, and I can't remember a time since fifth grade that I didn't feel shame about my body. I'm a Christian and have been praying for answers for years and years, but it turns out that I was just praying to God to help me serve my idol of beauty so I could finally be happy and free. I missed the point entirely. I've been in the false religion of "dietism" and used it to measure my rightness or wrongness. I have served another God and been in bondage I didn't even know I was meant to be free from. . . .
>
> Now, when I am tempted to fixate on my appearance, or feel ashamed that I'm not beautiful, I pray, "God, captivate me with your glory, your beauty, and your body. Not mine." And, "Lord, please help me to be brave enough to resist my culture's answer for this. Help me apply your gospel to my weight and my body image." Your blog is helping me do this. It's helping me dream a bigger dream, a dream past being smaller, a dream of really being free from the idol of beauty and the shame I've had no matter what size I've been from 10 to 20.

As I shared in my story, I prayed the same prayers as Mindy. "Dear God, help me stay on this diet," and "Dear God, please make me thin!" were a constant whisper. As Mindy put it so well, these prayers were to serve my interest, not his.

I bristle when I hear statements like "God made every woman beautiful!" and "You are enough!" used to appease a woman's body image struggles. The problem lies not within these answers; they may be fine for some. But to the heart struggling with body image idolatry, these answers will never satisfy because the question is rooted in worldliness. The woman struggling with her appearance doesn't wonder if she's beautiful enough to achieve God's purpose in her life—she wonders how she ranks in our culture's beauty contest. Her motivation is wrong. Or, as James says, she asks out of her worldly passions, not a passion for God.

Worldliness wins when we forget why we were created. When we believe and pursue looking good in a swimsuit as much or more than God's purpose for our lives, we've been sucked up into its vacuum.

The trickiest part of battling beauty and body image idolatry? Seeking a better physique may actually be a good thing. It may feel like you aren't doing anything wrong. For example, losing weight may be exactly what you need to get healthier, live longer, or fight disease. Similarly, exercising can be really good for you and have a positive effect on your overall well-being. But when diet, exercise, or any other avenue we pursue to change our outward appearance becomes of the utmost importance, we are trapped in worldliness, and it shifts into idolatry.

Finding the balance between pursuing health goals with vigor while not allowing them to become idols proves challenging. People often ask me about balance. As I mentioned in an earlier chapter, finding balance isn't the best goal.

We don't need balance; we need properly ordered affections.

A Greater Affection

I had to pay $19.99 to meet my husband.

Yes, it's true. I met my husband on eHarmony. You've seen the commercials. Yes, we were almost in one. Our audition video exuded lameness—to the point that when they called and asked us for a second audition, I was sure it was a prank. Alas, we weren't chosen to record the ads. *So close.*

Somehow, whatever algorithm it is that eHarmony uses to match people worked so well on us we fell in love—almost immediately. Sure, now I understand that those early feelings were really infatuation, not love, but convincing me of this a few weeks into our dating relationship would not have been possible. Something strange began to happen to my eating habits as our new love blossomed. Maybe you've had this happen, too. For a solid six months I didn't need to diet. I stopped thinking about my next meal. I didn't come home from a date and finish off the bag of Doritos and the mint chocolate chip.

I was too full for mindless eating. Not full of food, though. Rather, I was full of something else. Love!

We'd go out to dinner, and I could barely finish my plate. It makes me laugh to think of how often we split something—like a regular-sized burrito. One year later, my husband would have gotten the "stink eye" (as he calls it) had he recommended we split a burrito that small. When I met him, I found something I loved more than food. Him! *He* consumed my thoughts. *He* motivated my actions. I had a greater affection—my boyfriend.

Sir Thomas Chalmers was a Scottish minister who preached during the early 1800s. One of his famous sermons and writings was titled *The Expulsive Power of a New Affection*. In it, he speaks to the challenge of following a moral code and addresses how an individual can best break a bad or sinful habit. To paraphrase his main idea, he states that there are two ways a man can attempt to steer his heart away from the love of the world and things of the world. One way is to demonstrate that the world's way is meaningless—so that your heart no longer deems it valuable. The second is to give the heart a new object of affection. The latter is often more effective.[2]

According to Chalmers, if you try to drive out that old habit—say, emotional eating—by simply telling that annoying pattern that there is no longer a place for it, the habit may slowly creep back into the empty space. So, whatever you use to replace your bad habit has to be really, really good. Finding victory in our body image battle requires us to find an affection more worthy and more captivating than the illusion of what beauty promises. Jesus must become our greater affection.

I completely understand how amorphous that may sound. I struggled when told that I needed to just "crave God" more than I craved brownies. I had absolutely no idea how to do that. Truth is, brownies are really delicious and seem quite satisfying in the moment.

Some would look at my story and say I had an eating disorder (and according to the definition, I certainly did). On a deeper level, I had a heart disorder. And until my heart could be repaired, neither my body image obsession nor my eating could ever be truly healed.

Why Didn't Those Christian Diets Work?

For those of us who struggle with body image, I've found that many resources for gaining health—both Christian and mainstream—overlook the depraved state of our hearts and skip right to health strategies. Even Christianized dieting advice becomes ineffective unless it is rooted in the gospel.

Here's more of my friend Mindy's story:

> I have done every diet and diet/Bible study known to man, and the whole time I really believed that the problem was what I saw in the mirror—and the ugliness I saw in the mirror was there because I couldn't pull it together and just force the restriction and physical punishing that was required to get and remain thin.

Mindy, don't you know your body was made to be the temple of God? Look what you've done to it. You've ruined it. You were fearfully and wonderfully made and you ruined it all. You're an ugly mess now, especially that belly and neck of yours. You're fat and gross and what does that say to the world about God? Apparently you love French bread more than your beloved Jesus. You're a pig and you won't just stop eating. Jesus died for you to be free from sin and you aren't trying hard enough. Stop being a glutton. Other people do it all the time. Haven't you got any resolve or self-respect? Just imagine what people think of you. You know, you wouldn't feel this way if you could just be thinner, prettier, and more together.

I'm sorry you had to read that harsh quote from my mental life, but I include it because I know I have sisters out there who will feel a pang at reading their own thoughts in mine. We have a common enemy who spews this kind of evil at many of us. This line of reasoning has been reinforced all over culture and in many words from important people across the years of my life. I am emotional writing those words up because although I see now how horrid they are, I believed them, and I'm fighting not to be embarrassed by them now. What cruel shame. What an unbearable burden and bondage.

You see, I didn't know I had a body image issue. I thought I had a fat issue. I didn't know I had a shame issue. I thought I had a dieting issue. I didn't know I had an idolatry issue. I thought it was a failure issue.

I prayed and apologized to God for what I'd eaten, how much I'd eaten, or how I didn't exercise enough on such a constant basis that I really thought he was as concerned about my thinness and dieting as I was. I thought he was as fed up with me as I was. I thought his first priority for my sanctification was for me to win the battle on the scale so he could use me to the degree he wanted to. I thought he was waiting on me to clean myself up in response to what Jesus did for me on the cross. I thought it all depended on me. I did fasting and cleanses, and diets and starving, and massive amounts of exercise. I also did stress eating, comfort eating, and no exercise, and then I would throw in the towel and try to forget how bad I was, until the shame crept up again and I started all over. That sounds super healthy right? Clearly not. I thank God he hasn't left me there.

As Mindy so eloquently put it, our problem isn't a lack of willpower. We don't have fat, dieting, or failure issues—we have idolatry and shame issues masquerading as body image woes.

Letting the Gospel Speak to Our Body Image Idolatry

There are two types of people in this world. Those who load the dishwasher carefully and those who do not.

I'm in the latter category. I generally rinse things off before I put them in, but I'm no perfectionist. Just a second ago, I emptied dishes I had (obviously) loaded and found stray pieces of dried grapefruit woven through the silverware holders. Sometimes I find knives still coated with peanut butter or cups still stained with coffee. My solution is always the same. I just put them back in the dishwasher and run it again.

This drives my husband crazy. He begs me to put the item in the sink, spend two seconds scrubbing, and then put it back in so it will really be clean.

Nice concept. But seriously, who has time for that?

So I run that same stained knife through the cycle, over and over again. Hoping that one of the washes will eventually work.

When Jesus saves us, he desires to clean us fully. Yes, sanctification (the process of becoming holy) takes time. Though we don't completely transform overnight, his goal is for us to be cleansed from the past and stain-free through his blood. He cleans us thoroughly before putting us in the dishwasher of sanctification. He removes the stains so we don't have to bear the marks of sin any more.

I knew that Jesus could set even the worst of sinners free. I saw how, for so many, salvation meant a transformed life. But it wasn't until I uncovered the sin in my body image struggles—until I clearly saw my own idolatry and propensity toward worldliness—that I realized just how much I needed God's grace and how I needed the blood of Jesus to cover my sins, too.

The gospel certainly has something to say to our body image issues.

The gospel speaks directly to our hearts and calls us valued, no matter what shape our bodies are in. His truth speaks to our souls and says we are loved beyond (what our hips) measure. The gospel confronts our messy lives and says, "I loved you messy. Now, let me help remove the rest of that stain." To the voice of the enemy who whispers in your ear, "They'd all love you if you weighed less," the gospel specifically says, "No, the most important person loves you already—just as you are."

I had never understood the gospel in this way before. I had no idea how Jesus dying on the cross had anything to do with my tendency to obsess over the scale.

Turns out, it had everything to do with it.

I thought I just needed to try harder. Yes, it was "God and me," but a whole lot of that equation rested on me and my own strength.

As Mindy said in her story, I thought God would use me and love me more once I got all my junk together in the food and weight department. I read that he could take away my body image shame. Since it hadn't happened yet, I assumed that was a byproduct of him answering my prayers for a better body.

Friend, if you claim Christ as your Savior, if you say you are saved, I want you to ask yourself, honestly, if you've really allowed him to rescue all of you. Do you believe he can help you with your body image issues? Do you believe he can replace your affections with a greater affection for him? Do you believe that you can find true and transcendent joy and peace in him alone, or do you still think that maybe one of your idols can deliver?

And do you believe that Jesus's sacrifice was enough? Have you acknowledged just how powerless you are to change yourself, but how powerful he is to do a mighty work in your heart?

Don't be sorta saved. Believe your Savior can save you from your body image struggle, too.

This is step one: Let the gospel redeem your body image. Examine what salvation means to you using the questions in the Heart Exercises below before you move on to step two.

Chapter Mirror

We sometimes misunderstand the role salvation plays in our freedom. In the case of body image struggles, we get lost looking for salvation to come from weight loss or from the other ways our idolatry deceives us into thinking it will come. This worldliness sneaks in and taints our motives and true purpose. We lose our first love and misplace our greatest affection in our quest for a better body. The answer lies in finding true salvation, accepting his grace, and understanding how the gospel has something real and relevant to say to your body image battle and in keeping your affections in order. We must also understand that we are powerless to change ourselves—we'll never have enough willpower to get it right—yet through Jesus's sacrifice, we can be healed.

Heart Exercises

Read Romans 1, Romans 8:20–22, Romans 5:4, and James 4.

1. What does salvation mean to you? Do you believe you are saved?

2. Read the passage from Romans 1. In what ways do you think you may have gotten caught up in worshipping the created instead of the Creator? Do you struggle not to desire worship yourself (i.e., to have other people admire you or think that you are beautiful)?

3. Read all of James 4. In what ways do you think your battles mirror some of the conflicts James mentions in this passage? How would you define worldliness as it relates to your body image struggles?

4. Do you think salvation includes freedom from body image struggles?

5. What do you think of the concept of affections? What do you think your greatest affection has been recently? Do you believe your affections are in order?

6. In Romans 15:4 and Romans 8:20–22, what does Scripture give us? What does Paul say we are struggling with now and for what purpose? How does that relate to our body image battle?

7. In what ways have you tried to do it on your own—beat your body image battle with your own strength? Have these ways worked? Why or why not? How do you think this chapter will help you change your strategy going forward?

Memory Verse: "For freedom Christ has set us free; stand firm therefore, and do not submit again to a yoke of slavery" (Gal. 5:1).

Notes

[1]Timothy S. Lane and Paul David Tripp, *How People Change* (Greensboro, NC: New Growth Press, 2008).

[2]Thomas Chalmers, *The Expulsive Power of a New Affection* (Minneapolis: Curiosmith Publishers, 2012).

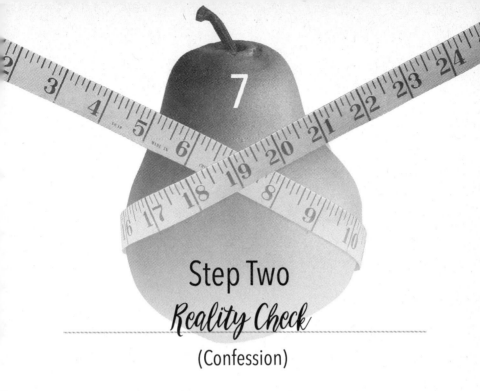

Step Two
Reality Check
(Confession)

"When our Lord and Master Jesus Christ said, 'Repent,' he willed the
entire life of believers to be one of repentance."

—MARTIN LUTHER, the first of the Ninety-Five Theses

"Whoever conceals his transgressions will not prosper, but he who
confesses and forsakes them will obtain mercy."

—PROVERBS 28:13

Pregnancy never slowed me down. I continued to teach fitness
classes well into the third trimester during all four of mine. Sure,
Braxton-Hicks contractions captured me and forced me into a
horizontal position by dinnertime most evenings. But I refused
to act disabled. After all, didn't women centuries ago work in the

fields all day and then just squat down and deliver their own babies? If they were that tough, surely I was, too.

Then there was the day I needed to get out my winter maternity clothes. I have limited drawer space, so I only keep the current season's clothing within reach. (And since I live in Texas, the current season—for what seems like nine months of the year—is summer.) My off-season (read: cold weather) clothing resides in large Rubbermaid bins stored above the hanging clothes in our closet. I mentioned to my husband a few times that I needed him to get that container down for me; he just hadn't had a chance to do it yet.

I'm not a tall person, but if I stand on my tiptoes, I can usually maneuver the bin I want out to the edge of the shelf and then brace myself for it to fall into my hands. After a decade of living single, I reasoned that retrieving this bin, all by myself, would be no big deal. I've taken care of toddlers. I've simultaneously carried two fussy kids up the stairs for naptime, each one kicking on either side of my seven-months-along, round baby belly. Catching a plastic box filled with sweaters? *Not a problem.*

I cleared some space on our closet floor just in case the bin flew by me. Then I started scooting it closer and closer to the edge. The container teetered on the rim of that board—ready to come down—when my then one-year-old decided to toddle into the closet looking for me. Distracted from my primary task, I yelled at him (one hand still braced to catch the bin) to move out of the way. He responded by just standing there, staring, as if he didn't understand English.

I moved my hand to motion him out of the room—maybe sign language would work. Within a second the bin crashed down. On its way, it caught another box filled with old purses. (Note: clean out the closet. *Someday.*) Both boxes bounced off my head and knocked me to the ground. My little guy got hit by a flying black, formal clutch but generally fared much better than his mother. He stood there staring at me as I sat on the floor, watching those little cartoon birdies spin around my head.

When my husband returned home, I informed him (matter-of-factly) that I almost died that afternoon trying to get my stretchy long pants down from our closet. His response? "I would have done that for you. Why didn't you just wait for help?"

"Because I didn't need help. I'm not an invalid, I'm pregnant," I retorted.

"Next time, just wait."

Perhaps I did need some help.

"Cause of death: struck by a heavy bin of winter clothing" is not how I want my obituary to read.

Can We Admit It?

Sometimes our biggest obstacle to finding help is admitting we actually need it.

For example, if you are trying to lose weight or maintain weight loss, experts will tell you to weigh yourself regularly. (Although when I know my heart is wrestling my body image idolatry, I take a break from the scales for a certain time period.) You don't need to be compulsive. But weighing yourself at the same time once or twice each week helps keep you on track. Why? Because viewing the scale on a regular basis keeps you grounded in reality. An additional ten pounds can't surprise you because you'll notice that number creep up slowly, digit by digit. It's sound advice that keeps us out of one arena that our heart really prefers to dwell in—denial.

Just like those extra pounds, sin can creep up on us. It may start with just a small step off the course God has for us. Then we wake up weeks or months later, snared deep in a trap we didn't even see. I'd argue that very few Christians premeditate having an affair, developing an addiction, or even marrying someone who isn't a believer. Yet one date leads to another. One flirty email leads to an inbox full. One night of soothing your pain with a substance leads to repeating that behavior. Again and again.

For those of us bound by the sins related to our body image battles, confession is the place to start. We need to raise our hands to God and say, "Yes, I admit it. I have a problem. I need your help. I'm stuck here." Alcoholics Anonymous made famous the twelve-step program to recovery, and experts agree these steps can aid recovery from other addictions. Most people are well aware of the first step. It's the joke someone will inevitably use in a circle of new people asked to introduce themselves. "Hi, I'm Heather, and I'm a brownie-aholic." Don't let the importance of the confession involved in that statement get lost in the punch line. We need to admit our weakness, admit we need help, before we can find a way out.

When I researched the twelve steps, I found it interesting that steps one through five are all about confession and surrender. Step one says, "I'm addicted." Step two follows with, "It's so bad that I know only God can help me." Step three essentially states, "Hey, God, I need your help." Then steps four and five are about searching our hearts, finding other areas of sin, and also admitting them to God, ourselves, and other addicts.

Alcoholics Anonymous Steps 1–5	
Step 1	We admitted we were powerless over alcohol—that our lives had become unmanageable.
Step 2	Came to believe that a Power greater than ourselves could restore us to sanity.
Step 3	Made a decision to turn our will and our lives over to the care of God as we understood Him.
Step 4	Made a searching and fearless moral inventory of ourselves.
Step 5	Admitted to God, to ourselves, and to another human being the exact nature of our wrongs.

Something transformational happens when we acknowledge, with words, the ways we grieved God and others. We take the first step toward the freedom God intends us to have from the struggles (and addictions) that bog us down.

Confession offers really great news for everyone who suffers with body image. If you only consider your body image struggles to be "normal girl problems," there is no remedy. You carry that sack of "normal girl problems" around with you forever—like still carrying your stocked diaper bag when your children enter elementary school. But if we call our struggles sin—by clearly identifying the ways our hearts have been distracted by worldliness and other idols—then we find a remedy. God's cure for sin is confession. For my friends who—like me—tried every diet, exercise program, and spa treatment to find freedom from these issues, this should come as really great news.

Why Confession?

In 1 John 1:9, the Bible says, "If we confess our sins, he is faithful and just to forgive us our sins and to cleanse us from all unrighteousness." Though some people believe this to be a one-time confession of sins at the point of salvation, I believe Scripture calls for a continual confession of sins. The Lord's Prayer in Matthew 6 demonstrates that we should ask God to forgive us as frequently as we ask for our daily bread.

Right before this oft-quoted confession verse, John clarifies *who* is in need of this type of regular confession. The verses in 1 John 1:7–8 read, "But if we walk in the light, as he is in the light, we have fellowship with one another, and the blood of Jesus his Son cleanses us from all sin. If we say we have no sin, we deceive ourselves, and the truth is not in us." The followers of Jesus walk in the light, and yet we must continually go back to God and tell him ways we failed to keep his commands.

I'm not sure who said it. Somewhere along the way, as we prepared to plant a church and go into full-time ministry, we heard a more experienced minister say the following words: "Keep short accounts with God." The reason for this sage advice? When you regularly confess the ways you err, you stay closer to the course God has for you. In other words: weigh yourself regularly. Confession resembles your regular weight check. If you go a few months without stepping on that scale, pounds sneak up on you. But if you check in on a regular basis, you'll distinguish them sooner.

Confession in Community

Theologian and martyr Dietrich Bonhoeffer wrote in his book *Life Together* that confession triggers a breakthrough to true community. Sin "demands" us to stay out of community. We withdraw, so it isolates us. He asserts that the more alone our sin makes us, the greater its power grows.[1]

Bonhoeffer pointed out that sin is only exposed by the light of the gospel. Since the confession of sin is made in the presence of a Christian brother, the last stronghold of self-justification is abandoned. The sinner surrenders; he gives up all his evil. He gives his heart to God, and he finds the forgiveness of all his sin in the fellowship of Jesus Christ and his brother.[2] Once you've confessed your struggle as sin to a fellow believer, you've released a great deal of the power it holds over you. You can no longer say, "It's okay. It's just my issue. I'll keep it hidden right here in this little space no one knows about."

You confess it out loud so that you can actually be free from it. Yet we fear others seeing our flaws. Don't believe me? Okay, how many times have you worn makeup or worried about what outfit you would wear in the presence of other women? Seriously! I do it because I want other women to think highly of me. I want them to perceive me as put together, not flawed. I don't want them to see the real me—the thoughts I hide with shame or the sunspots and scars concealed by my medium-coverage foundation.

The thought of someone knowing exactly what I'm struggling with and being close enough to say, "Hey, Heather, are you not eating tonight because you are dieting again?" or "Heather, why *won't* you get your picture taken right now?" scares me silly. I'd rather not have anyone call me out on issues like that. I'd prefer to keep it quiet so that when I fail I'm the only one who knows.

Don't I do a good enough job at self-condemnation? Do I really need to involve someone else? And that's when the Bible says yes. We do, for that very reason. When left alone, *all* we give ourselves is condemnation. Though we may fear criticism from other Christians, chances are they'll meet us with understanding. "I hear your struggle, but his Word is true and you are still valuable to him . . . and to me."

A Patient Father

For some of you, the thought of coming to a father and asking for forgiveness from sin feels daunting. Maybe your earthly father had a bad temper. The thought of telling him you did anything wrong terrified you. Or maybe you never knew your biological father, and you don't really have any frame of reference for relating to God as Heavenly Father. Perhaps you instinctively imagine a mean boss or abusive boyfriend, and you worry about God's reaction if you confess sin to him.

I want to encourage you that God is gracious with us. As we confront our sin, God deals with us patiently and lovingly. He is a good father, not a monster sitting in heaven, angrily tapping his foot on the ground, saying, "Any day now . . . come on . . . get it together."

Not at all.

Instead, imagine him as the father who stands on the far side of the room with his arms open wide and urges his one-year-old to take that long journey across, one wobbly lunge forward after another. The toddler takes a step and then falls. She gets up and takes two more quick steps before stumbling again. Still unsteady, she tries to find her balance and takes a few more steps, slower this time, until she gets almost close enough to touch her destination. With those outstretched arms just a few feet away, she turns into an Olympic speed walker right into the embrace of her father.

God graciously waits for us to come to him and confess to him our sin in this battle. He welcomes us home.

What Am I Confessing?

God our Father will show us where we fall short, if we ask him. Because most of our struggles are common, I find the areas we most often need to confess are the following: idolatry, covetousness, comparison, and humanism.

We've talked at length about idolatry and the ways we fall short of God's plan by replacing him and his kingdom for cheap, material, and worldly substitutes. So the most effective way to confess our idolatry is to first clearly identify the ways we commit idolatry. I have found a simple way to do this. Spend some time in prayer and ask God to help bring to mind things you may be missing. Take a pen and your journal and answer these questions:

- What can't I live without?
- What makes me crazy?
- What do I think about when I'm alone and all is quiet?
- What does my heart really, really long for?
- Who am I following other than Jesus?
- Whose opinion matters most to me?

The answers to each of these questions will lead you to the areas where your heart strays. I'd encourage you to confess to him every area of your heart's wandering. Lay it all out before him and bring it to light.

The interesting and potentially lethal thing about idolatry is its link to all of the other sins in which we find ourselves ensnared—jealousy, comparison, lying, stealing, adultery . . . you name it. In each of these cases, you can probably identify a root of idolatry that led the person into the deeper sin.

For example, we first need to deal with the idol of body image idolatry before we can effectively deal with our own struggles with comparison. If we can root out the fallacy of our idolatrous thinking—recognizing that a great figure and a beautiful face aren't sources of real salvation—then we become less likely to compare ourselves to other women. We can drop out of comparison's silent beauty pageant because we know where to find real life and joy.

This leads to a second main area of confession: confessing the ways we covet others. Simply put, when I covet, I desire what others have. It often indicates a lack of contentment on my part. One day, God revealed to me my own covetousness during a sermon on the Ten Commandments. The pastor read through Exodus 20, and at verse 17, he caught my attention with the list of some possessions a neighbor may have that we may desire, like oxen, sheep, or an amazing spouse.

On this particular day, my phone's Bible app had somehow defaulted back to the King James Version, and I noticed something peculiar. Right there on my screen, that list mentioned my neighbor's "ass." Of course, the Bible refers to a donkey. In that moment, God reminded me of something. Wishing I had a bottom as firm as Jennifer Lopez's was coveting just the same as wishing I had my neighbor's mule.

Ask yourself if you desire the things others possess more than the good gifts God gives you. Pose these questions to yourself and write down your answers:

- What do I long for other than Jesus?
- Do I have a stronger desire to have her abs, her booty, her high cheekbones, or her (fill in the blank here) than I do to follow Jesus?

Next (swallow hard here), you will want to tell the Father ways you've compared yourself to others. Confess to him those thoughts. Some you may never have said out loud, yet trying to measure up to her. *Or her. Or her.* It all falls into the realm of comparison.

Do you envy that person's size, shape, look, or life? Then, my friend, call it sin and realize that it needs to be brought to the light and confessed. Even though we may not know the person we've been comparing ourselves to (it may be a celebrity), we sin when we spend time wishing for someone else's life or despising our own in contrast. In an upcoming chapter, I'll spend more time on comparison and how damaging it is. For now, confess the ways you've followed someone else's race instead of running your own. Answer these questions:

- Who am I trying to be like other than Jesus?
- Who is it that I compare myself to most often?

Ways We've Bought the Self-Esteem Lie

Another area of confession you may need to release to him is buying into the lie of humanism. You might think, "Heather, this is a really weird one that I'm pretty sure I don't do." If so, write down your answer to these questions:

- Do you ever try to convince yourself that you are awesome (or good, or enough) without (or aside from) Jesus?

- Have you ever said you *need* something? Maybe you've even convinced yourself of the fact that you need (fill in the blank here).

Friends, so many of us hear so much junk on this whole topic of how to feel better about ourselves that we may need to cleanse ourselves from the wash of "self-love" and "self-esteem" propaganda. Even some of the self-focused stuff we've heard at church has to go!

Remember the personal pep rallies I held in my head before speech competitions? I think many of us do the same to bolster our self-confidence before we head out the door in the morning. We look in the mirror and think, "Nailed it." We feel confident for the day. What happens when our self-esteem runs out? How about those days when the image staring back from the mirror screams, "Have you seen your stomach? You may not want to go out like this!" Let's say it's that time of the month, humidity creates less-than-ideal hairstyling conditions, and your stress pimple has surfaced right smack dab between your eyebrows. How does self-love help us on mornings like this?

Someday we will fail, and those cheerleaders in our head that say, "You are *soooo* great! Go you!" will change their chant to, "Wow, you stink! I can't believe how lousy you really are!" You probably had this experience already. (I certainly have!)

It's so subtle how correct the self-love movement seems. There can't be anything wrong with loving me, right? "I have to love myself before I can love others," they say. Sometimes they even use the Bible to encourage us to try these humanistic strategies. With a slight wording twist, we Christians are instructed to stare in the mirror and in awe of how awesome God made us, or we are to "see ourselves" as incredible because that's how he sees us. We use our culture's #Iamenough without thinking twice as we superimpose human wisdom on to God's Word.

This is why we stay stuck.

We want to praise Jesus and ourselves at the same time, on the same level. I just don't think that's possible or biblical. Allow me to explain.

The Bible's Not a Self-Esteem Manual

I speak to MOPS (Mothers of Preschoolers) groups regularly. I love telling these communities of newer moms that there is hope for their body image struggles.

But on one particular day, right before I got up to give my hour-long talk, a mentor mom from their group was introduced. The group's leader said she'd asked this mom to speak for a few minutes on the topic of her choice. A sweet woman in her sixties walked to the podium and shared that she would talk about body image, too. Sirens went off in my head; I tried to remain calm. I anticipated what she would say because people in church usually say the same things on this topic. So I braced myself. I could hear it coming. (*Sigh . . .*)

Then she said it. All of it. She repeated every line that I've ever heard spoken in church about the body image issue and our struggle with it. I was touched by her courage. She spoke openly about the details of her personal struggle. But I was saddened by how, after she preached the standard lines about how God made all women beautiful and it's what's on the inside that counts, she said the following. "We'll probably always struggle with this. I have."

I knew I needed to follow that delicately. I appreciated her truthfulness, though I wondered how many women have battled the body image issue for most of their lives and accepted the fact that hope will always elude them. To some degree she was right. This side of heaven, life will never be idyllic. We will always strug-gle—as the book of James delineates—with worldliness. But the Bible offers us encouragement. It tells us that freedom (even on this issue) *is* attainable. Nowhere does Scripture say that God's will for his women is that they wrestle with a desire to look physically different. It's not true that this is the one battle we can't find victory in on this earth. The problem is that we turn the Bible into a self-esteem manual.

The Christian platform on the topic of body image consists of three main tenets. I'll list them as follows:

- True beauty is on the inside.
- Your body is awesome because it is the temple of the Holy Spirit (1 Cor. 6:19).
- God made every woman (physically) beautiful (in her own unique way). Because you are fearfully and wonderfully made (Ps. 139:14).

Sometimes different Christian sects throw into the mix some of Peter's words about refraining from wearing jewelry or worrying too much about our clothing. For the most part, this sums up all Christian women ever hear on the topic of body image. Through the decades I spent in Christian schools and evangelical churches (of all denominations, including nondenominational) and through everything I have read, researched, and studied, these are the main and often the only "Christian" answers I've seen given.

Think I'm wrong? Just Google it. Lots of content is dedicated to these topics.

The fact is, most of us know these verses (and truths) already, and they don't help. The reminder that God made me beautiful—stretch marks, cellulite, and all—doesn't cure my struggle. My personal war on this topic runs much deeper than these three Christian clichés address.

Candidly, the real problem is that we use these verses (and truths) to glorify ourselves instead of God. We look for affirmation of our own greatness in God's Word and miss how the Bible points to God's glory, not our own.

Psalm 139:14 is a great example. The verse says, "I praise you, for I am fearfully and wonderfully made." When we read it with emphasis on the words "I" and "wonderfully," it sounds like it was written to accentuate our own human greatness. As one comedian said, I think "the em-*pha*-sis is on the wrong sy-*lab*-le." In other words, I don't think David intended for us to read it this way.

The psalmist wasn't writing to build himself up. David was such an amazing worshipper that he once embarrassed his wife by dancing in the streets praising God (2 Sam. 6). He wrote these words to exclaim his awe for an incredible God who could make us so intricate and amazing. In fact, when David feels down, you can see what he often does through the Psalms. He exclaims the awesomeness of his Creator—not his own! This seems to contradict what culture would tell us to do when we feel low: "Just remember how awesome you are!"

Psalm 139:14 is not a verse to remind us of our own greatness. *No. It's about God's greatness.* Are our bodies amazing in design? Yes. But let's get real. We didn't have anything to do with that. Give credit where credit is due, right?

The Bible brims over with ultimate truth that speaks to our body image battle. It's just not all found in the verses most often used to address this topic. Instead, it's found in the gospel of Jesus Christ and in the story of God's plan to redeem us. We need to recognize that we are nothing apart from our Savior—he is the source of our value. Though telling women they are already "enough" sounds nice, the truth is we aren't "enough" without him. Apart from him I can do nothing, as Jesus says (John 15:5).

Here's another way to think about this: I don't think God looks at us and is impressed. God looks at us with great love—a father's love—and compassion and mercy! Yes! But we are his creation; *He* is our Creator.

This reminds me of when my budding artists decide to draw me a picture. I love my children so much that I encourage them and proudly display their artwork on our art wall. Yet I know its value is limited. Though it's important to me, if I try to take it to the Louvre in Paris and insist they hang it next to the Mona Lisa, I may get hauled off to the mental institution.

We're the same way.

Yes, we are made in the image of God, the *Imago Dei*—more valuable than any of God's other creations. A unique combination of body and soul that sets us apart from the animals and the trees and even the angels, we are extremely valuable because of who our Creator is and how he created us. But *he* is the one worthy of worship for the masterpiece of humanity.

Author Jay Adams discusses many of the problems with the ways that even Christians have accepted humanistic viewpoints in his book *The Biblical View of Self-Esteem, Self-Image, and Self-Love*. The Bible, he says, shows us a huge gap between Jesus Christ and us in order to challenge us through justification and sanctification to try and close the gap. He argues that accepting ourselves, delighting in ourselves, and focusing on our self-worth damage the process of sanctification, as they make us satisfied with who we are right now. Why do I need to change if I'm already great?[3]

Have you bought into the self-love lie? Have you told someone that she needed to love herself before she could love her husband or children well? That's not exactly biblical, either. Have you thought that your problem in your marriage was that you just don't love yourself enough?

Our bodies are temples of the Holy Spirit, yes. We don't worship the temple, though. We *use* the temple to worship and bring glory to God. Instead of staring in the mirror harder to find something to love about ourselves, we need to tilt the mirror up and start reflecting our Savior. Freedom comes not through self-acceptance, but through self-forgetfulness.

And Then There's Gluttony . . .

I can be completely full after a satisfying meal and still eat dessert. And not just a bite or two of dessert, depending on what it is—like if I'm at the Cheesecake Factory and indulging in the Reese's Peanut Butter Cup Cheesecake—I'll keep eating long after I'm full. I'll keep eating until it's gone. You can't waste cheesecake that good, right?

No one wants to use the "G" word, ever. I don't think I've heard a full sermon dedicated to the tender topic. (I guess it takes a thin pastor to preach on gluttony?) But I would be remiss if I didn't mention it as something that you may need to confess, if it applies. Not every woman who struggles with body image also struggles with gluttony. I do, and so I'm guessing some reading this do also. Gluttony, simply put, is eating too much for the wrong reasons. It's a sin just the same as drinking too much (drunkenness) or sleeping too much (laziness). It's funny how the Bible really does give great diet advice. Moderation is the key!

Figuring out exactly where the gluttony line is—that's more like folding fitted sheets, hard and certainly not neat. Do you have to figure out the precise number of calories you need for a day and track what you eat carefully so as not to cross it?

I don't think so.

Like all other sin issues, gluttony reveals a heart issue. The question is more about how you use the food versus the specific number of calories or bites you eat. Do you run to the food for comfort? Confess that to Jesus and realize your comfort comes from him. Do you turn to food to help with your stress, anxiety, or worry? Confess, repent, and acknowledge that Jesus carries your burden better than those chocolate chip cookies. Do you use food to feed your hungry soul? Then confess that, and realize that what your soul starves for contains no wheat, dairy, nuts, or soy.

Just like all other bad habits, our tendency to overeat is more about a misuse of food—as a substance we hope will numb our pain or heal our hurt—than it is about overindulging in a Thanksgiving feast. Uncovering the heart behind your food struggles isn't easy. It will be a process. But begin the process by confessing these struggles to Jesus (and a close friend, too) if you want to start on the path to freedom.

This is step two: **Confess the Sin to Find Freedom.** Use the Heart Exercises below to explore your views on confession and uncover any areas of un-confessed sin in your life.

Chapter Mirror

Confession is vital and necessary for finding freedom from the body image struggle that entangles us. To find release from our sin, we need to confess to God and to others. We commonly need to confess wrong actions or wrong thinking in these four major areas: idolatry, comparison, covetousness, and humanistic thinking (buying into the teachings of self-love). If overeating is a personal struggle, then confess the sin of gluttony and ask your patient and loving father to give you his grace and help in this arena.

Heart Exercises

Read James 5:13–18.

1. Do you see confession as a necessary part of the process of reconciliation with God and healing? Why or why not?

2. What do you think you may need to confess specifically in the four main areas of struggle?

   Idolatry: What do you chase after, other than Jesus?

   Comparison: Who do you emulate, other than Jesus?

   Coveting: What do you long for, other than Jesus?

   Humanism: Do you tend to think you are awesome in your own strength at times? Or do you believe you are too bad or unworthy to receive his grace? (Remember that high self-esteem and low self-esteem are both the same pride issue.) What practical ways can you think of to retrain your mind on this issue?

3. Read 1 Chronicles 16:8–36. What do we hear David do in this passage? What does David say about the people's idols in this passage?

4. How can you tell if your eating crosses the line into gluttony? Is this a struggle for you?

―――――――――――――――――― ∾ ――――――――――――――――――

Memory Verse: "If we confess our sins, he is faithful and just to forgive us our sins and to cleanse us from all unrighteousness" (1 John 1:9).

Notes

[1]Dietrich Bonhoeffer, *Life Together: The Classic Exploration of Christian Community* (New York: HarperOne, 2009), 87–88. The German edition was originally published in 1939. The English translation was first published in 1954.

[2]Ibid.

[3]Jay E. Adams, *The Biblical View of Self-Esteem, Self-Love and Self-Image* (Eugene, OR: Harvest House Publishers, 1986), 77–79.

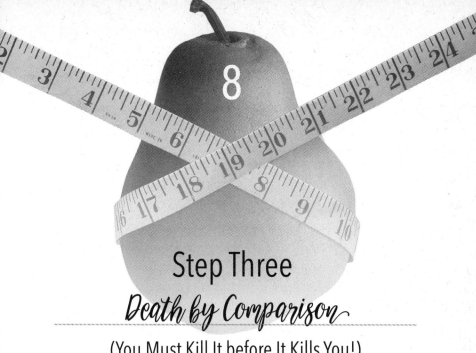

Step Three
Death by Comparison
(You Must Kill It before It Kills You!)

"Comparison is the thief of joy."

—THEODORE ROOSEVELT

Everything in the picture looked amazing.

Flawless holiday decor framed the background. The table, beautifully set, featured every type of delectable Christmas treat you could imagine. I would have mistaken it for a photo taken straight from the December cover of *Better Homes and Gardens*. The headline could have read, "How to Host the Perfect Holiday Party."

The image wasn't from the cover of any magazine, though. No. I saw it on Facebook.

Christmas Eve was a busy day in the home of this pastor's wife. But somehow amidst the chaos, I managed to give my newsfeed a quick scroll. I scrutinized every aspect of that photo while barking commands at my children. "Come on, get your shoes on!"

"No, not those shoes. Find your dress shoes. Hurry! We need to go!"

I clicked my phone off and threw it in my purse. But I couldn't get my mind off that picture. *That's what Christmas Eve should look like*, I thought to myself.

As the garage door closed, I visualized the shambled state in which I left my house. Decorations were the backdrop to a very messy kitchen. My dining table stood full of paper plates littered with leftover Mickey Mouse chicken nugget ears and ketchup dollops. Because my children struggle to remember what napkins are for, my once-clean Christmas tablecloth now had nice smears of the red condiment beside every place setting.

Yes, quite the Christmas Eve feast at our house. (Ketchup is a vegetable, right?) To my credit, some half-decorated sugar cookies were shoved into a snowman tin on the counter (festive, I know). But there was no spread. Nothing pretty enough to photograph and post on social media.

I battled condemning thoughts. "You should do better. Your children deserve a nice Christmas Eve feast like that. What kind of memories are you building for them?" I schemed ways I could make up for our dinner when we got home from service. *Maybe I could thaw out some of the leftover hors d'oeuvres from last weekend's Christmas party. I could create a table like that. Of course, I'll have to wash the tablecloth first. As soon as I get home, I'll . . .*

To excuse my perceived holiday Mom-fail, I consoled myself with reminders of how hard it is to get four children dressed (in Christmas best) and out the door without my husband there to help. (Seems the pastor needs to go to church early, always!) I patted myself on the back for having my own hair and makeup done. I managed to get out of my yoga pants and red sweatshirt ensemble and into a more holiday-appropriate outfit. I was doing okay.

But I could do better.

The image of her perfect holiday burned in my mind. Instead of listening to the sermon, I plotted how my buffet table would look next year. My family needed a beautiful Christmas. I should be that kind of mom—a better mom. If only I was skilled at things like arranging food to look nice on serving platters.

The picture struck me so powerfully that I hadn't even noticed who posted it. I saw it and immediately started comparing myself to her without even looking to see who "she" was. Only hours later, when I scrolled back through that Facebook feed, did I read the name of the woman responsible for that picture-perfect holiday table. It was a friend who was alone on Christmas Eve. In fact, this friend's life was turned upside down as she faced the dissolution of her marriage. Her children were with her soon-to-be-ex-husband. She stayed home, alone on this night, preparing for them to come and spend the holiday with her tomorrow.

Of course, none of that backstory could be found in the Facebook post. No caption on the picture read, "I'm really lonely today because the kids are at his house, so I'm putting all of my energy into making things nice for tomorrow." Or, "Divorce is the hardest thing I've ever gone through. I hope I can make the other parts of our celebration beautiful even though the most important part—the family part—will be messy."

The image did not tell the whole story. This is just one reason we must always ask the question, "Compared to Who?"

She Still Struggles

Would it shock you if I told you that even your friends who look perfect struggle with their body image? In fact, I've found that women who always appear like they've got it together may actually struggle even more than those who can't seem to pull off perfect very often (or very well).

Many of the emails I get from readers of my blog share that they've suffered alone. I hear comments like, "No one knows how much I worry about my weight and appearance." Readers confess that, although most people think they have nothing to "worry about" with the way they look, the battle consumes them. They are always working to be different, thinner, more toned, or more beautiful.

Earlier in this book I shared with you the words of Cameron Russell, the Victoria's Secret model who confessed that models are the most insecure women on the planet. Some of you read that and still think, "I don't care. If I looked that way all my problems would be solved." I've thought that before. Comparison is just another way that we believe the body image idolatry lie. We take our idol, a beautiful body, and we project it—in all of its glory—onto a person. She possesses our idol—physical beauty—and so we falsely believe her life resembles a happy, pain-free, and nonstop carnival ride.

But is it true?

Hardly.

In this chapter, I want to share with you some strategies for uprooting comparison in your life. Although I know it's easy to default to a place of envy when you see someone who looks like she has it all, I hope that through this section, you will see how comparison deceives us and steals our contentment.

Let's break down the truth about comparison.

Comparison Will Kill You: Is It All in Our Heads?

Pinterest is incredible for getting ideas. It also causes many women great dissatisfaction. I am not at all crafty, and when I see the DIY projects that moms and their children (allegedly) work on together all day long, I feel inferior. When I witness the way these

Pinterest-perfect women decorate their homes (or cupcakes), can change their fireplace mantel decor for each season, and then make all-natural freezer meals ahead for the next forty days, I feel lazy and incompetent.

I'm lucky that we get our Christmas decorations up and down each year. One year we simply forgot to put our lights up. (I felt so guilty that the pastor's house looked like the only one on the block not celebrating Christmas!) I took the holly wreath off my door the day after Valentine's Day. (It was red, right?) The thought of hanging Easter or Fourth of July decor is not even close to making my to-do list.

I have a friend, Jennifer, who recently became a stay-at-home mom. She anticipated spending her days working through these pin-worthy projects and teaching her children a second language. I laughed out loud when she shared that secret. Not to make her feel bad, of course, but because I knew her expectations were not boarding the same shuttle bus as reality.

She shared her frustration. "Heather, I just don't have time to do anything I thought I would." I smiled in response and told her that if she could make dinner and fold some laundry while caring for her newborn and preschooler she should consider that a good day. If she could accomplish those two tasks without the assistance of the Disney Channel, she should consider that a *really* good day.

"Seriously? That's such a relief. I thought I was failing. I thought there was something wrong. I thought I just wasn't very good at this mothering thing, and it was killing me."

She found herself stuck in a place where she felt stressed and unable to enjoy her new life as a stay-at-home mom. Jennifer constantly compared the realities of her new position with an elusive and unrealistic picture in her head of what a stay-at-home mom's life looks like.

Friend, isn't that what we do when we battle to be beautiful? We have an image in our heads of what life would be like if only we could go into the store and have anything we pick off the rack look good on us. We are confident that more joy awaits if we could just get flatter abs or sculpted arms. We compare ourselves to the woman who has what we think we want, and so we work (and work, and work) to do better . . . to catch up!

We strive (and strive, and strive) to reach our goal. Until we get tired. And then, for some of us, we eat. (Others avoid food. Not me, though. I eat when I'm frustrated.) Then we feel bad about the eating (or not eating). Then we feel depressed. Then we take some time off to wallow in our misery. And then somehow we get distracted and manage to pick ourselves up out of the pit. Soon we start striving all over again.

That's not freedom. That's life in the cage of comparison. Comparison chains us to our body image problems. Even once we've confessed the sin of body image idolatry and received Christ's forgiveness, comparison still lurks. Like a commercial for your favorite candy, she suddenly appears to lure us into craving what beauty idolatry offers. "Wouldn't you be happier if you looked different? Being beautiful sure has worked out well for her. Or, maybe you should consider trying to lose a few more pounds."

Comparison lies about where we'll find true contentment. She cheats by glossing over details like the fact that the thinner woman isn't necessarily the happier woman. And she steals.

She steals our joy.

Comparison beats us down. It keeps us always feeling like we aren't doing well enough. Sure, in a feeble effort to appeal to our ego, comparison may point out some progress we've made or identify an area where we excel. But then she'll pack an almost invisible punch as she lists other shortcomings or prods us to just do a little better.

The mental obstacle course comparison puts us on is exhausting. Though we may have small victories in the comparison game (thinner than her—ten points), we end up in despair when we face loss (not thinner than her—minus twenty). The up and down roller coaster of thoughts—"Today I feel good about myself because at least I'm better than she is," and then, "Today I feel bad about myself because I saw her"—isn't fun (or healthy or Christlike) at all.

It's death.

Comparison puts me in a position to spend a lot of time thinking about one person. Yes, you guessed it. Me! "How does she compare to me?" is the filter through which I view the world. With a posture of comparison, I find myself in constant competition—I always need to know where I stand.

If you wonder why you feel insecure, think about just how precarious a place it is that comparison forces us to reside. Like trying to walk on a giant jellyfish, you aren't sure when the standard will squish up or down. (And at any time it could sting you!) Never knowing if you're winning or losing, that's frustrating. You can gain ground and feel like you are progressing only to have the rules change. Imagine how women who were trying to fit into a perfect size 10, like Marilyn Monroe in the1950s, felt when Twiggy became the new, skinny standard of beauty in the mid-1960s. Culture's standards change. Comparison makes the struggle to be beautiful downright cruel.

Adding a Storyline

I'm a huge fan of the Olympics, and I love cheering for team USA. It makes me feel so patriotic. During my single years, I had the opportunity to go to the Atlanta summer games and the Salt Lake City winter games. Talk about dreams coming true! I was going to make the most of my Olympic experiences.

Though I'm somewhat of a sports fan, I realized that there is something vastly different about watching the Olympics in person versus viewing them on your living room flat-screen.

In February of 2000, I bought tickets to attend the finals of the bobsled competition. They weren't cheap, but I didn't care. I thought it would be so exciting to stand right there on the mountain and experience the thrill of seeing them race for gold.

There was only one thing I hadn't calculated. Watching bobsledding live is absolutely boring. In fact, *watching* bobsledding is really a misnomer. You don't watch a bobsled like you watch an airplane take off or watch athletes race around a track. No, when you have a ticket for a bobsledding competition, you stake out one particular spot along the expansive track. Then, about every six minutes, you hear a loud rumble and are vaguely aware (as you see a flash of color pass before you on the track) that the next competitor has taken a turn.

In between runs, there's a lot of downtime, a lot of time to stand there, think about how cold it is, debate whether a third cup of hot chocolate qualifies as excessive, and wonder if you'd possibly have a better view from anywhere else on that mountain. Memorable? Yes. I can say, "Been there. Done that." But I didn't leave with a passion for the sport of bobsledding. Nor did I leave with a connection to any of the actual athletes. I couldn't see them as they flew by. In fact, I didn't even catch most of their names.

Juxtapose this with sitting in front of your television watching the very same competition. In between runs, you hear the stories of the athletes and their families. The screen cuts to images of the driver as a seven-year-old in his native country with his homemade sled. The producers create a compelling (and almost fictitious) storyline that engages you. The camera zooms in on the competitors' faces as they prepare for their run. You follow the coverage of the sport not because bobsledding interests you, but because you want to cheer for this team or that athlete whose story touched your heart.

One of the biggest reasons we struggle with comparing ourselves to other women is that we don't get close enough to follow anyone else's storyline. It's very easy to become indifferent at an event such as the Olympics when you don't know this competitor from that one. But, once you know more about the people themselves, you become invested. If you struggle with comparing yourself to the women around you, I'd encourage you to really get to know them. Until you learn their stories, you aren't viewing them as fallible, struggling, and human. In fact, you may be objectifying them.

I know, you probably thought objectifying was something that only men do to women. But women can do the exact same thing to each other. When we look only at someone's outward appearance and value (or devalue) them for that alone, we too fail to see them as human. We miss that the woman we compete with needs love, too, and we view her as an object. (It's kind of like that line from the old movie *Notting Hill* where Julia Roberts's character stands in front of Hugh Grant and says, "I'm just a girl, standing in front of a boy, asking him to love her.")

We often do this with celebrities we desire to emulate. We forget they are real women and see them only for their physical beauty. But the image doesn't tell the whole story. Though we may not actually be able to get to know who they are (and their storyline from the gossip page may not actually be helpful to our cause of viewing them as more human), we are called to love them, too. All you have to do is read the headlines surrounding the perfect-looking woman on the cover of the gossip magazine to be reminded that although she has beauty, she still struggles with depression, anxiety, and relationships.

When it comes to women in our circles, I've also been amazed at how quickly "sisters" in Christ will use words like "hate" when it comes to a woman who has a faster metabolism than she does. Few statements irk me as much as this one does. Saying, even in a joking way, that we "hate" thinner or "prettier" women perpetuates body image lies and feeds the beast of comparison. Even joking like this harms and reveals what's in the heart of the joke-teller (Luke 6:45).

Shouldn't we stop objectifying, judging, "hating," and writing off others we perceive as better off in the looks arena? We need to remember that they still struggle.

So many times the woman who looks like she has it all together is the woman who desperately needs a friend because she feels like she's falling apart. I know because I was that woman. The more messed up I felt, the more compulsively put together I became. The more caught up I was in my body image struggle, the longer I would spend on my hair, makeup, and outfit before leaving the house. (I would often change clothes at least ten times and then redo my hair to better suit my outfit.) The woman people saw at church on those days may have looked polished on the outside, but she was a complete disaster on the inside.

I would also ask that you pray for that other woman. Committing yourself to pray for another person softens your heart toward her. After a while, it's hard to dislike someone you're asking God to bless. When we know each other's stories, it becomes a whole lot harder to compete. We begin to realize that we aren't racing against each other. Rather, we are each running our own races, facing our own obstacles, and trying to find a pace we can sustain.

Freedom Isn't Elusive

I have young children and, therefore, we watch movies—lots and lots of kid movies. We don't have cable. So, aside from PBS, popping in a movie was the coping mechanism of choice while having four babies in the course of four and a half years. I know each of their funny lines, and, regrettably, sometimes I lie in bed at night singing their catchy tunes.

A few years ago, Veggie Tales and Barbie put out movies with the same plotlines and similar titles. While the veggie version of "Princess and the Popstar" tells the story with cute little feminized carrots, Barbie plays both title roles in her version of "The Princess and the Popstar." Both stories were loosely based on an old Mark Twain story, *The Prince and the Pauper*. The plot cleverly reveals what happens when you get caught in the trap of comparison. In the Barbie version, a princess believes her life would be more exciting if she led the life of a popstar. Meanwhile, the purple-haired popstar is looking out her window dreaming about the royal life of a princess.

And then there's the song—the way-too-catchy song that goes with all this daydreaming. It's called "I Wish I Had Her Life," and the chorus chants how living in someone else's shoes would surely be better. In fact, the lyrics go beyond just calling out the luxuries of living a "better" life; the song uses another word that grabbed my attention the first time I heard it. The song echoes, as each girl sings, "I wish I had her life, then I would feel so . . . free."

Free?

Isn't it interesting that what we truly long for is not a better life—but a freer one?

Freedom. That's what we really want. We innately value freedom more than wealth, stardom, or a royal title. The song appeals to a woman's deepest desire—one she may not even recognize—that is, for someone to save her and set her free. Our tendency is to chant this mantra (often subconsciously) as we compare ourselves to others. We look at her thin frame, shapely legs, or beautifully styled hair and think, "I wish I had her life . . . then I would be so free!"

I've been there. Many of my closest friends over the years have been taller and thinner than me. My bridal party photo is a gaggle of tall, thin girls, average-height me, and my petite sister-in-law. I once believed that if I were just a little taller and my body mass had a few more inches upon which to distribute itself, then life would be easier. If I could be taller, then I could be thinner, and then I would be free from my "miserable" life of dieting, exercising, and trying to change my body's shape—just like my tall friends.

Or so I thought.

But it's just the comparison trap. And, as both the Barbie and Veggie Tales movies reveal, life isn't always better in someone else's two-inch pumps. We mistakenly believe that freedom comes when we find a way out of the troubles that personally weigh us down. We forget that other women face troubles of their own.

I hope you'll stop believing comparison's lie. Being someone else is not where freedom can be found. Being yourself in Christ Jesus is where you find true freedom. "Where the Spirit of the Lord is, there is freedom" (2 Cor. 3:17).

Freedom and grace. We all need grace.

Grace Isn't Fair

Free advice for those who attend potluck functions: if you are trying to watch what you eat, do not sign up to take brownies. Or, at a minimum, take them to your social event uncut. I'm sure I'm not the only one who struggles, so this is solid advice. It's impossible to cut brownies and not sample the scraps. (You know those huge hunks of crumbs that are left stuck to the knife when you try to make the pieces even in size? *Yum.*)

At our house brownies go fast. Of course, everyone always wants the "big" one. Never, not one time, have I heard one of my children say, "Here, my sister can have the huge piece, and I'll take that small one over there. Thanks, Mom." The debate centralizes around justice and equity. It has to be fair. It's not right if someone gets a super-sized brownie, and I don't.

Sometimes our hearts cry foul when we feel someone else has been blessed in a way that we haven't. We get jealous of the fact that she can eat junk food and not gain weight. We envy how her body curves in the right places or how clear her complexion looks. We make comparisons based on our own sense of fairness. No one ever had to tell my children that it was fair for everyone to have the same size brownie. They deduced this on their own.

In the same way, when caught in the trap of comparison, our "It's not fair" alarms start to blare at a decibel that drowns out all other reasonable thoughts.

- It's not fair that she doesn't have to skip dessert.
- It's not fair that she doesn't have to straighten (or curl) her hair.
- It's not fair that she doesn't have to exercise.
- It's not fair that she can look good in that style of jeans.
- It's not fair that she blah, blah, blah . . .

We forget that life's not fair. More, we forget that grace isn't fair. We forget to be thankful for that fact.

When Paul told us to run our race toward the prize of the high calling of Jesus Christ, the image he paints is not one of a track with a bunch of women giving themselves whiplash as they constantly check to see how they are doing compared to everyone else running the course. Do you know what happens to Olympic athletes who turn their heads to check their pace? They lose the race. Of course, you never see trained athletes do that. They know better. They know to fix their eyes on the prize and run their own race.

We need to run our own races, too.

We should measure ourselves only against Jesus. His standard doesn't fluctuate like our culture's standard of beauty. We can rest secure in where we stand with him and confidently work to grow more like him, knowing he is unchanging. I've learned that the best way to combat comparison is to keep my focus on him, receiving his grace daily. He shows me where and how I need to correct my pace. No one else is worthy of comparison. And there is no one else with whom I can compare myself and strengthen the relationship rather than weaken it.

Know Your Purpose

Yesterday I sat at the airport waiting to board a plane to Miami for an annual pastors and wives retreat. My husband and I made it through the security strip-down and found a seat near our gate. As I sat there, I observed hundreds of other travelers rush to catch their flights. Some pulled suitcases; others lugged around their children (and their Disney-themed backpacks) just to get there faster.

I noticed one thing as I sat there in front of the sign that said "Flight 303: Miami." All the people in an airport know where they are going. Once through security, each person carries a ticket for a specific destination. No one strolls through the airport looking over all the gates to decide which flight to take that day. No one sizes up the crowd getting on a certain flight and chooses, at that point, to go to that destination, too.

Now, sure, on the way to our gate I may have jokingly pointed out the flight leaving for Hawaii and recommended we board that plane instead. But, even in my jest I wouldn't have lingered there. My purpose for that day included travelling to Miami, not Maui. To become distracted by that flight or to sit there and whine about the fact that all those people get to go to Hawaii while I only get to go to Miami would have been downright foolish.

My plea to you, dear friend, is to know your purpose. Understand that God has given you a unique objective on this earth and all of the talent and abilities you need to accomplish that purpose. Be as determined to fulfill God's will for your specific life as a person trying to catch an airplane. Though you may not always feel like you know where you are going, believe that God issued you the right ticket. He gave you exactly what you need to get there. Stay focused until you arrive, trusting that God will lead you along the varied path to a destination he's chosen for you. Don't let the distractions of where others are headed slow you down. Know that what you look like may or may not play a role in that purpose, but it certainly will not keep you from accomplishing it.

I once heard Nick Vujicic speak. He was born without arms or legs but has an incredible ministry—he travels the world preaching and has led thousands to Jesus. He said he once asked God, "How can a man with no arms or legs be your hands and feet?" The unstated answer: God gave Nick, physically, everything he needed to fulfill God's purpose for his life. He did the same for you, too.

Purpose cures comparison.

Step three for overcoming your body image battle is to break out of the comparison trap. Free yourself from concern over what she's eating, wearing, driving, weighing, lifting, or flying to. Stop singing, "I wish I had her life" or pinning pictures of the girl with the abs you want. Remember, the image doesn't tell the whole story, and you have a unique purpose God equipped you to fulfill. Keep your eyes on your own race.

This is step three: **Cut Out Comparison.** Use the Heart Exercises below to explore what Scripture says about comparison, and then spend some time this week reflecting on ways comparison may be having an impact on your life.

Chapter Mirror

Comparison keeps our eyes off God and his plan for our lives. The lie of comparison tells us that others have it better than we do, but we forget how the image never divulges the backstory. Everyone— including those we compare ourselves to—struggles. We must also remember that both life and grace aren't fair, but we should be grateful for that. Every woman runs a different track with different hurdles. We must run our own races and spend less time comparing our progress to that of others. We must compare ourselves only to Christ. Having another woman's looks or life isn't the path to freedom. Freedom is only found in him. And no matter what we look like, he designed us with a great—and unique—purpose.

Heart Exercises

Read James 3:14, Philippians 2:3, and 2 Corinthians 10:12–13. Then answer the following questions.

1. What common themes do you see in these three passages? Do you believe comparison helps or harms your body image struggles?

2. What specific areas tempt you to compare yourself to others?

3. How do you think that getting to know others' "storylines" would help you in the comparison struggle?

4. Is comparison a "normal girl problem" or a sin? Why?

5. In what ways do we harm ourselves by engaging in comparison?

6. According to 1 Peter 1:22, how are we to love each other? How do you think comparison harms our relationships with our sisters in Christ?

7. Read Genesis 29. What lessons do you think we can learn from Leah? What do you think about the fact that God didn't make Rachel and Leah equally beautiful—physically? Is this difficult for you to accept? Why or why not?

———————————— ∾ ————————————

Memory Verse: "But if you have bitter jealousy and selfish ambition in your hearts, do not boast and be false to the truth" (James 3:14).

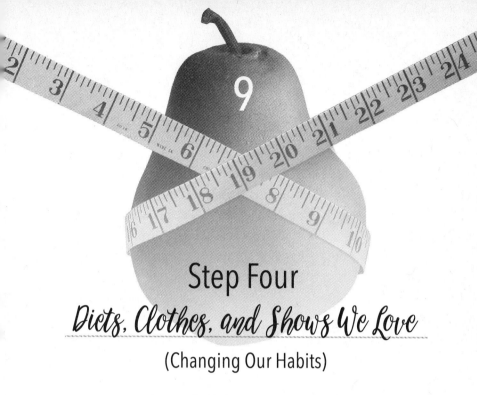

Step Four
Diets, Clothes, and Shows We Love
(Changing Our Habits)

"A change in bad habits leads to a change in life."

—Jenny Craig

No one can make my hair look as good as my hairdresser does. Kara works magic with a flat iron and round brush. In less than two hours, she can make roots and split ends disappear, and she can turn my funky curls and frizz into straight, shiny, and smooth-looking locks.

She's brilliant.

So I *should* always leave the salon feeling like a celebrity. My hair will not look that fantastic again for at least six to eight weeks. I *should* hold my head high and smile because it feels so good. But a strange thing happens at the beauty salon. As I sit there under the dryer, a voice calls out to me from a basket below—it's the magazine basket, filled with the latest issues of *Vogue, Us Weekly,* and *Glamour.* Headlines like, "Dress to Look 10 Pounds Lighter" and "The Four Foods You Should Never Eat" whisper directly to me. "Hey, just spend a few minutes reading me. You need the information I have. It'll be okay to take a quick look."

So I bite. I grab the magazine and start flipping pages. I see image after image of touted perfection. I notice her incredible figure. I see her sculpted abs. I covet those clearly defined muscles in her arms. While one side of my brain starts thinking of ways I could add more weight lifting to my routine to get arms like that, the other side spots a super cute outfit and starts plotting when I could get to the store to pick up a skirt in that length and color.

A few pages later, I realize I need a new lipstick color. Mine is so last season. I flip another page to find out my jeans aren't in style anymore. I quickly notice my out-of-date shoes. Denim cuts and heel widths have changed. Again. A few more pages and I'm convinced my happiness really does hinge on losing another ten pounds. By the end of the magazine, I hurry to get out of that salon because I have some serious exercising, dieting, and shopping to do!

Oh yes, and then there's my hair—the hair that I should now love and be exuberant about. It's not actually good enough anymore. Why didn't I have her cut some cute bangs? All those celebrities in *People* have them now. Why didn't I go bolder with the highlights?

I create my own world of discontent.

You Are What You Eat

Though it's difficult, losing weight isn't really a great mystery. (Unless you battle thyroid disease or other health obstacles like I do.) Ultimately, no matter what diet or exercise program you try, reducing the number on the scale comes down to making healthier food choices and having your exercise output exceed your food input.

Food has to transform its place in our lives from friend and comforter to nourisher. We have to feed our body for energy, out of hunger, versus using food to fuel our emotions or soothe us. I could counsel you on many habits surrounding food, exercise plans, and dieting. I could spend an entire chapter giving you my best tips and tricks for changing the way the outside of your body looks.

The problem with that is twofold. First, it would be a waste of your resources and time because chances are every tip I could give you is one you have read or heard somewhere else in some similar form. (When Solomon said in Ecclesiastes that there is "nothing new under the sun," he spoke with keen insight into the future cyclical nature of America's diet and exercise trends.)

Second, you could use my tips to achieve your best body ever and still struggle with body image. (If you still aren't convinced this is true, please go back to Chapter Two and read and watch Victoria's Secret model Cameron Russell's story—again!)

What we put in our body's system matters. *Yes.*

Should you try to eat healthy and take care of your body? *Yes. Of course.*

But for the purposes of this chapter, we won't talk about what you put in your mouth. Instead, we'll talk about what you put in your head and the habits generated out of those systems of belief. Many women I meet are a lot more aware of what it means to eat healthy than what it means to have body image healthy habits. They know their fat grams and calorie counts but don't see the dangers that come from what their mind consumes.

There are ways that we mess with our brains and open the doors to be defeated. I think there are practical things you need to do in conjunction with this book to see and feel like you are making progress. This chapter is difficult because we'll talk about ways you need to change your habits. We'll get real about the actual things that you do every day—things that, in some cases, you may have done all your life—that you probably need to stop doing if you want to find victory here.

Ouch!

Here's what I want you to remember: freedom will come from all these steps together. Not just this one. But if you skip this one, you may never find relief.

Media Mayhem

When I speak, I love asking women in the audience this question: If you knew that your husband struggled with lust, would you buy him a subscription to *Maxim* or *Playboy* magazine for his birthday? A nervous giggle followed by a stubborn indignation fills the room. Unanimously, the women yell, "No!"

I affirm their decision. Of course a sane Christian woman wouldn't do that. Looking at those images would trigger thoughts in your man's mind that are neither healthy nor holy. Looking at those images would encourage him to sin. In fact, if he confessed to a struggle with lust, you'd likely rid your entire home of anything that could contribute to his struggle. You'd install accountability software on his computer and ask him to destroy any pornographic movies or magazines. You'd insist he get rid of it all so that he could start down a road to repentance and recovery from this harmful habit.

So, friends, this is where it gets tricky. But I have to ask you, just like I ask every audience I speak to: How many times a day do you look at images of other women that trigger thoughts for you that are neither healthy nor holy? Although pornography use is on the rise among women,[1] I don't just mean porn. I mean those fashion magazines that stare you down in the grocery store checkout line or those clothing catalogs you love that are delivered to your mailbox each week. I mean your favorite TV show (*The Bachelor*—ladies, now I know this hurts some of you), "chick flick" movies (where everyone looks stunning), or romantic novels.

What you consume matters. Just like you are what you eat, you are heavily influenced by what you watch, see, read, and hear. For some of you, this will be a tough one. But it's so important. In most cases, we have complete control over what media we consume, yet we put very little time or thought into how healthy and holy these choices are. We fool ourselves with the same lie that I believe at the hair salon: "Just a little bit won't hurt."

Yet it's never true. A little bit of poison still makes a noticeable impact.

I cancelled all of my magazine subscriptions almost a decade ago. Part of the reason: I realized that having those images around my house wasn't helpful for my husband. My main motivation at the time was probably misguided. I thought I was safeguarding my marriage by making sure my husband didn't see anyone more beautiful than me, but as a bonus, living magazine-free helped me break out of the comparison trap.

Even if there was some redemptive content in the publication, the ads in these magazines often shouted a louder and more harmful message about my value and what beauty offered. If you can't look at images like this without having unhealthy ("Look at her body, I'm so fat!") or unholy ("I wish I looked that good in a bathing suit. Then I'd be happy") thoughts, then you need to change your habits, too.

When my husband and I married, older friends advised us that watching too much TV might not help us adjust to life as a couple. So we didn't have cable. We watched movies when we were desperate for home entertainment, but we eliminated the possibility of sitting mindlessly for hours flipping around stations pumping messages we didn't need to consume. It likely bettered our new relationship.

It's not just the images that harm us. Sometimes the plot lines do, too. They reinforce the lies we believe accompany beauty. We think that if we looked different, then we'd have a man who would do and say the same things that the leading man in the latest romantic tearjerker says and does. Even those nice stories—the clean ones with barely any kissing—can send us false messages about love and romance that send us into a spiral of comparison and discontent.

Many women suffer from romance addiction—something I believe harms our marriages. No woman who consumes a lot of romance virtually is able to enjoy her real-life relationship with her husband. Similarly, no man who consumes a lot of pornography is able to fully enjoy his real-life intimate relationship with his wife. (We'll talk about this more at the end of this chapter.) We buy media lies. We invite the beauty and comparison beasts back into our lives and find ourselves in the body image pit once again.

We need to ask ourselves some hard questions about the media we consume. We must search our hearts and honestly uncover the damage. It's almost ironic how so many of us who struggle in this arena would be very aware of how much junk food we ate, but not as aware of how much garbage we feed our minds. If you struggle with the way God created your body, ask, "Did I recently watch something or read something that I'm comparing myself to?" Pray for God to reveal the media message which caused you to struggle. Then be bold. Cut it out.

You'll survive without it.

Expect that, like an addict, you will miss it for a while. Expect it to hurt (for at least the first few weeks). In anticipation of your withdrawal process, don't leave that space empty. Where you used to fill free time with novels (which require your imagination to come up with pictures and can be just as dangerous as that NC-17 rated movie!) and *TMZ,* replace it with something better. Read your Bible, talk to a friend (not on Facebook—a real live person!), read a solid book on a topic that interests you, or watch or listen to a sermon. It will amaze you what redeeming the time you once wasted will yield in your life.

Psalms 119:37 says, "Turn my eyes from looking at worthless things; and give me life in your ways." His Word also instructs us to guard our hearts, for they are, as Solomon writes, our wellspring of life (Prov. 4:23).

Media is the chain that binds us to our body image battle. Take action and free yourself from its captivity. The idea that you *need* it is a lie. *You don't.* This doesn't mean you can never watch another TV show or see the latest blockbuster movie. A diagnosis of diabetes doesn't mean you can never eat another brownie, but I encourage you to treat media like junk food. Be careful about what you see and how much of it you consume.

Some of you still need to be convinced to stop this habit. I understand. I know that some media seems to give us a connection with friends, gives us something to talk about at the office, or (we think) gives us pleasure. But I'd encourage you to look at this data from JustSayYes.org.

Facts about Media Influence on Body Image[2]
After viewing images of female fashion models, 7 out of 10 women felt more depressed and angrier than before they viewed the images. (Rader Programs)
80 percent of women who answered a *People* magazine survey responded that images of women on TV and in the movies make them feel insecure. (Rader Programs)
69 percent of girls in 5th–12th grades reported that magazine pictures influenced their idea of a perfect body shape. (National Association of Anorexia Nervosa and Associated Disorders)

Another thing to consider—even if you think you aren't impacted, your daughter (and son) may be. Studies show the more reality TV a young girl watches, the more likely she finds appearance important.[2] When a mom tells me that she and her daughter enjoy watching *The Bachelor* together, I want to cry. Literally weep. I can't think of a worse thing to fill my daughter's head with than the notion that she is in a beauty contest against a bunch of celebrity-model-looking women for the attention of one man. That sets her up for disaster.

Retrain Your Thoughts

"Look at how puffy you look."

"You can't leave the house looking like that."

"I wonder if I can lose ten pounds before . . ."

These were the voices in my head a few years ago. I focused on them, answered them in their folly, and allowed them to consume me. I needed to change the way I spoke to myself!

The Bible tells us in Romans 12:1–2 to be transformed by the renewing of our minds. What interests me about these verses is that transforming our minds is connected with how we prepare our bodies to be presented to God. Read the whole passage here:

> Therefore, I urge you, brothers and sisters, in view of God's mercy, to offer your bodies as a living sacrifice, holy and pleasing to God—this is your true and proper worship. Do not conform to the pattern of this world, but be transformed by the renewing of your mind. Then you will be able to test and approve what God's will is— his good, pleasing and perfect will. (NIV)

Our self-talk often nurses our sin. And just like a hungry monster, most of the time we feed our body image challenges with negative self-talk. We say things to ourselves we'd never say to another human being because these comments are so straight-up mean!

Please don't misunderstand me. I don't think our answer lies simply in pepping ourselves up with positive thoughts of our own utter awesomeness. (If you haven't clearly gotten that message from the other chapters in this book, reread them.) We don't need greater self-love or self-esteem. We need greater Christ-esteem. We need to know how awesome he is. Retraining our mind means we change the way we see ourselves, and then we talk to ourselves as Jesus would, not as we did before he transformed us.

If you believe condemning thoughts about yourself—*You're no good. You're fat, and no one will love you. You don't deserve love*—you should know without a doubt that Jesus doesn't believe this about you. These lies from the enemy will keep you in the pit if you allow them to.

Instead, 2 Corinthians 10:5 instructs us to take our thoughts captive in obedience to Jesus. Picture yourself as a comic strip character with a thought bubble over your head. Every time a message that contradicts what God says about you enters that thought bubble, you get to become a rodeo star. Take a rope and lasso the words out of the bubble and throw them off the page.

But that's often not enough. If you leave the bubble empty for too long, another thought will pop in. Chances are, it won't be a good one. To fight it, you need to replace the thoughts with a more truthful thought. Here's an example. If you think "I'm not valuable," lasso that thought and replace it with, "Christ dying for me gives me infinite value." Or, "If I could only lose this weight, then I wouldn't be so miserable." Lasso and replace with, "My joy and identity are not found in my weight. I will keep working to get healthier, but God isn't disappointed in me, and he accepts me because of his sacrifice."

A good exercise is to write down negative thoughts as you have them. Then spend time searching the Scriptures to find the antidote. Through this process, you will start to build an arsenal of thoughts to combat the lies the enemy brings to your mind.

Dare to Stop Dieting

If you are a chronic dieter like I was, let me encourage you to work on changing your patterns. The main problem with diets? They end. They start on Monday (or "tomorrow"), and they end whenever you can't take it anymore. (Or when a friend shows up at your door with a bag of Ghirardelli chocolates!)

Nothing with a start and stop date ever offers you permanent change. Dieting sets you up for a roller coaster of beginnings and endings. Diets make you feel in control, because you choose the program. But in reality, the diet controls you. You can submit to it for a time period, and then you rebel.

An article in the *Annual Review of Public Health* analyzed data from the most popular and successful diets of the decade, and they reached this conclusion. No one diet works better than another diet. Unable to recommend any diet over another, they made the following recommendation that, paraphrased, goes like this, "Eat real food, just don't eat too much."[4]

How's that for a diet plan?

I understand that you may read this and legitimately need to lose weight. Let me encourage you; it's okay to get healthier. But compulsive dieting becomes a habit, and in some cases an addiction, and it's not the answer. If you know you must lose weight (maybe a doctor asked you to for health reasons, or you know that you feel healthier and more comfortable closer to your optimal weight range), then I advise you to focus on your heart first and *then* work on changing your eating habits so your weight loss will last. In many cases, people who lose weight gain all the weight back in a few years.[5] I think this is due, in part, to their hearts never changing.

This isn't the only reason you should stop dieting, though. I believe you will never find ultimate weight loss "success" until you resolve in your heart why you *believe* you need to weigh less.

- Do you want to weigh less because of health risks?
- Do you think weighing less allows you to feel more accepted and loved?
- Do you want to shrink your size because it's slowing you down?
- Are you trying to match your body shape and size to some unrealistic ideal?
- Are you striving to become more like the "old you" without giving yourself grace for the ways your body has changed, grown, and performed (babies, hello)?
- Are you content to work on your weight loss until it's complete, or do you have a time period in mind by which you need to lose the weight?

Muse over these questions. Journal about them. Write the first things that come to mind. Often that reveals your heart.

In some cases, the answer may be all of the above! The scales at the doctor's office signaled trouble, but your heart still wrestles with the notion that life would be completely different—and better—if you weighed less. Granted, feeling healthy is better. *Yes.* Being at a healthy weight is not a bad motivation or goal, inherently. But solidifying your love for and desire to look to Jesus for your happiness instead of a thin body is where you will find freedom. Not when the scale says 135 pounds.

With your heart in the right place and health as your motivation for weight loss, then, and only then, would I recommend you talk to someone, like a nutritionist or doctor, to come up with a personalized plan for you. In this way, it *won't* be like going on another diet. Instead, it should feel like the first step to change your lifestyle (and habits) to create a new pattern. You may experience days where you can stick to the plan perfectly and other days where you deviate a bit, but either way you don't bear the guilt and shame of going off the diet or feeling like a failure.

Distinguishing a diet from a healthier lifestyle plan is like comparing religion with the gospel. Religion gives you a set of rules you must do to be accepted. If you mess up, you can think of yourself as "bad" and a "failure." Religion says obey the law, and if you can't get it right all the time, then you can't stay in our club. Then there's the gospel. The gospel takes the act of salvation, and it puts the burden somewhere other than on you—on Jesus. He paid the penalty for our sins so that we could be accepted. Now, as his followers, we are in the process of sanctification. We do what he commands out of obedience based in love. The guilt and shame vanish. We want to follow the guidelines because we know they benefit us and because we know the One who created the rules cares deeply for us.

For most compulsive dieters, this mindset shift should feel freeing.

Enough with Overexercising

Spinning is an exhilarating forty-five-minute ride on a stationary bike. On average, you can burn between 500 and 700 calories in just under an hour if you do it correctly with enough resistance added.

One August evening, the spin room felt steamy after a great ride. A woman in the back stood up from her bike to stretch and immediately started to fall sideways. A friend caught her and helped her off the bike and onto the floor. My thoughts raced—my first real emergency situation as an instructor. I frantically searched my brain to remember if it was three short breaths every twenty seconds or two short breaths every thirty when giving CPR.

I asked another rider to get her some water. She took a few sips and started coming back to life. My first question was, "When did you last eat?" Her answer—breakfast. It was after seven in the evening. Her friend at the next bike chimed in. "Yes, she was working outside all day before she came here." Fortunately, I always carry fruit (fruit-*flavored*) gummy candies in my bag for quick glucose (or for fussy children). This woman lacked the calories or sugar in her system to make it through that workout. I was lucky she didn't pass out while on the bike and really hurt herself.

I wish I could say that this kind of situation was rare. But it's not. Many in group exercise classes are trying to lose weight, so they don't eat before they come, or they don't eat enough to do strenuous exercise. Then I see people who abuse their bodies by exercising way too much. They don't have large amounts of weight to lose, but they watch reality weight-loss shows and decide to do two classes in a row and then run on the treadmill or lift weights.

Yes, exercise benefits your body, but it does have a limit, and that limit isn't to be taken lightly. Below I've listed a few ways you can tell if you're overexercising[6]:

- Exercise leaves you exhausted instead of energized.
- You experience the blues.
- You have a short fuse.
- You can't sleep or can't seem to sleep enough.
- You have "heavy" legs.
- Your muscles stay sore for days at a time.
- You get sick easily, or it takes forever to get over a cold.

If any of these apply to you, take heed. You likely work at too high of an intensity when you exercise, or you need to take more rest days in between workouts to allow your body to recover.

I encourage you to examine your heart with these questions:

- Why do you feel like you need to work out so much?
- Are there other things you could or should do with the excess time you spend at the gym?
- Do you derive worth and value from how much you're able to lift or how well you perform in the gym?
- Is being an "exerciser" or "athlete" an important part of your identity that you would be afraid to lose?

Check your heart and make sure exercise hasn't become idolatry. If that statement sounds unfamiliar, I encourage you to go back to Chapter Six and reread the section on identifying idols.

My Closet Addiction

I had a rule during my single years. It wasn't written down or anything. But I followed it faithfully.

I bought a new outfit for every first date.

It wasn't until my last-ever first date that I broke my rule. I wore something already hanging in my closet—a pink cardigan sweater set and a denim skirt. Apparently no connection between having a new outfit and getting a second, third, or fourth date actually existed. *Who knew?*

I share this story to reveal what a clothes maniac I once was. I spent a lot of time (and money—though I *am* a clearance rack only kind of girl) on clothing. I never needed a mall app of any kind. I spent enough time there to know that place backward and forward. Clothes mattered to me. *Too much.* An important ally in my fight against my body, they helped me look thinner and feel more confident. (So I thought at the time.) When my clothes failed, I felt like a failure.

If you struggle with body image, you may also have a troubled relationship with clothing. Maybe your closet overflows with outfits you thought you needed to get you through special occasions or modern fashions that didn't really turn out to be your style.

Pray for God to free you from clothing. Okay . . . that came out wrong. You don't want to live in a nudist colony. But God can free you from basing your daily worth on what you wear. I think his purpose for you transcends always needing the right outfit to affirm your value. He can help you feel secure in a much more comfortable way than Spanx (and all of the other IBS-inducing undergarments that make you look ten pounds slimmer) ever will. He wants for his daughters to look nice and reflect him, but he never desires us to obsess over our threads (Matt. 6:26).

And then there's the whole "M" word.

I hate to even mention the word modesty because so often we interpret the word to mean plain, unfashionable, or frumpy. Let me assure you, that's not where I'm heading as I broach this subject. The simple truth is that sometimes we use our clothes to help market our body because we've been competing with others in the arena of body image. We spend so many years believing that we find our worth in the way our bodies look that we learn to use clothing to accentuate the "goods."

Let me encourage you—you can wear stylish clothing that fits well while being modest. Modesty is more about your heart than your exposed skin. What motivates your clothing selection? Do you wear yoga pants to the grocery store because you think they make your butt look good and others will appreciate that, or because you just left the gym and this is your only chance to pick up some bread for the kids' lunch?

My best advice on the topic of modesty is twofold. First, when shopping, ask yourself: Why do I need this? Is the answer to feel good about your body? Then maybe you don't actually need it and you need to search for the truth instead. Second, ask yourself honestly: What do I want people to think when they see me wearing this? Is your goal to leave everyone thinking you're the hottest girl in town? Maybe you need to reevaluate. Is your goal for men (or other women) to think you have a hot body? Again, it may be time to stop and ask yourself if this coincides with what the Bible teaches.

Sex Won't Settle It

My head half-submerged in the rinsing bowl, I closed my eyes and tried to relax as Kara, my hair stylist, removed the foils woven through my freshly colored hair. I'm not an eavesdropper. (Correction: I'm not *always* an eavesdropper. I do "research.") But the lady reclining next to me started talking about going to the theater to see the second installment of the movie *Magic Mike*.

"Well, I felt a little dirty going into the theater," she confessed with a bit of a Texas drawl. "But my friends wanted to go live it up. One of them went out to the concession stand to get all her junk food so she could really enjoy it. But all I could think of was how these movies make me never want to eat again so I can be skinny enough to have sex that good."

My eyes popped open and met Kara's. She gave me a look that signaled she heard it, too.

Only hot bodies have good sex.

Or at least that's what she believes. It's not her fault—our culture propagates that myth. Of course, the way we feel about our bodies plays a role in the way we engage with others sexually. But the lie that only hot bodies have "good" sex destroys intimacy.

For the married woman, feelings of insecurity, shame, and body loathing can cause serious strain on the way she engages her husband in the bedroom. The single woman (or teen) may try to resolve the uncertainty about whether or not her body is "good enough" through sexual encounters outside of marriage. Sex and our body image share an obvious connection, and thus you may need to change some habits in this area.

First, to the single woman: stop having sex. I could have over-complicated that sentence but wanted to make sure you didn't miss it! You need to know that this isn't what God has for you. It may seem enjoyable now. I get it. But you're playing in a dangerous arena. It's sin, my friend. Consequences follow sin. Always. False intimacy that comes from sex outside of marriage only gives short-term happiness. It won't answer those questions you hope it will, either. Just because he thinks you're sexy enough to sleep with this week doesn't mean that he loves you the way Christ intends. He's already proving that he's not convinced God's ways are best. This will make your married life infinitely more difficult.

I know that's a hard truth. Your heart wants to know that you are beautiful and valuable and lovable. But sex isn't going to answer those questions for you in a satisfying way. In fact, there is an extremely high likelihood that the one you have given yourself to will go find another, and you will only be left with more questions and confusion. You can continue to find other partners to help you feel affirmed, but the results won't satisfy. Friend, please stop trying to fix your body image through sex. I mean sex of all kinds, not just the actual act. We can try to derive our value from sexual activity—outside of actual intercourse—that will leave us hollow and empty just the same as an actual sexual relationship would.

For my married friends, I want you to pray and ask God if you've made sex an idol. I did. I'll confess that to you with the hope it will encourage you to search your heart.

I thought my value to my husband was largely sexual in nature. If he didn't want me all the time, I felt unworthy. We fought about sex more than any other topic. I blamed my husband for my insecurity because he wasn't making me feel wanted enough. But it mattered little what he said or did because sex had become my idol—I pursued it to affirm my value, and it always let me down.

If you struggle with sex in your marriage, pray for God to show you the reason. All problems in marriage are a byproduct of two sinners in one relationship. Do not decide to blame your husband alone. Yes, he may be partially at fault, but allow the Holy Spirit to work on him. Work on your own stuff. Sort out the roots of your issues. Is your attitude about sex wrong? Do you suffer with guilt and shame from sexual experiences that took place before you were married? Do you withdraw from your husband because of other types of body shame?

Many marriages also struggle through one or both partners' lust issues. If your spouse looks at porn or watches soft porn on HBO or Cinemax, you need to know that this habit isn't about you. His sin is his sin. Most often, lust issues stem out of unresolved anger and control issues. The problem has nothing to do with your appearance. You could lose the weight, get the boob job, or have the body of a Victoria's Secret model, and he would still struggle. Pray for him. Seek counsel. Encourage him to seek accountability and support to get out from under the control of this damaging sin habit.

Similarly, if you are looking at porn, you need to get help. Don't wait. Confess it to a godly woman and seek good counsel. Porn takes the damage that normal media can do and escalates it immeasurably. You need to break free from your porn habit before you can find any freedom in body image.

Sex is important for a healthy marriage. I encourage you to talk to a biblical counselor if your body image battle has incited unhealthy habits and patterns in this area.

This is step four: **Change Your Habits.** Your path to body image freedom will likely require you to make some personal changes. Use the Heart Exercises below and explore which of your habits need a makeover.

Chapter Mirror

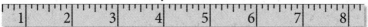

If you want to get healthy and stay healthy—spiritually—on the body image issue, then certain habits will need to change. The biggest probably relates to the media you consume, but other habits may include compulsions to exercise and diet, your relationship with clothing, and the way you engage in sexual activity. Identifying idolatry that has crept into each of these arenas helps free us from our body image struggles.

Heart Exercises

1. Read Psalm 119:37 and Romans 12. In what areas do you need to change your habits (media, dieting, exercising, clothing, sex)?

2. Habits are often hard to change because of our heart's idolatry connected to them. Have you been able to identify any false idols in your life that may be connected to any or all of the habits with which you struggle? If so, which ones?

3. Why don't diets work? Why do we put hope (and faith) in them so frequently?

4. Do you see a connection between the way you dress and your body image struggle?

5. In what ways do you think your view of sex connects to your body image battle?

6. List three things you can do this week to start to change your habits.

Memory Verse: "Turn my eyes from looking at worthless things; and give me life in your ways" (Ps. 119:37).

Notes

[1] Luke Gilkerson, "How Many Women Are Hooked on Porn? 10 Stats That May Shock You," Covenant Eyes (website), August 30, 2013, www.covenanteyes .com/2013/08/30/women-addicted-to-porn-stats/.

[2] "Self Image/Media Influences," Just Say Yes (website), retrieved July 5, 2015, from https://www.justsayyes.org/topics/self-image-media-influences/.

[3] Peter Christenson and Maria Ivancin, "The 'Reality' of Health: Reality Television and Public Health," discussion paper prepared for the Kaiser Family Foundation, October 2006, https://kaiserfamilyfoundation.files.wordpress .com/2013/01/7567.pdf.

[4] David L. Katz and Stephanie Meller, "Can We Say What Diet Is Best for Health?" *Annual Review of Public Health* 35 (March 2014): 83–103, www

.annualreviews.org/doi/abs/10.1146/annurev-publhealth-032013-182351 ?journalCode=publhealth.

[5] Priya Sumithran and Joseph Proietto, "The Defence of Body Weight: A Physiological Basis for Weight Regain after Weight Loss," *Journal of Clinical Science* 124, no. 4 (February 2013): 231–41, www.clinsci.org/content/124/4/231.

[6] Joseph Mercola, "7 Signs You're Exercising Too Much," Mercola.com, December 28, 2012, http://fitness.mercola.com/sites/fitness/archive/2012/12 /28/7-hidden-signs-of-overtraining.aspx.

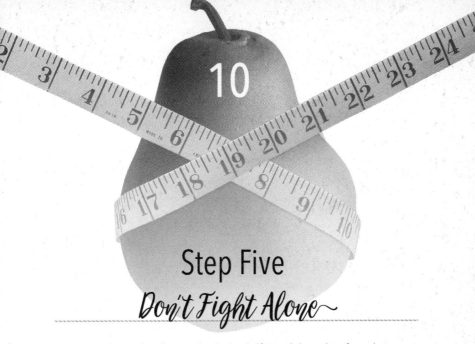

10

Step Five
Don't Fight Alone

"Sin demands to have a man by himself. It withdraws him from the community. The more isolated a person is, the more destructive will be the power of sin over him, and the more deeply he becomes involved in it, the more disastrous is his isolation."

—DIETRICH BONHOEFFER, *Life Together*

I remember well the day we all lined up in front of the mirror. We stood one in front of the other so we could solve it. It was the only way to determine a clear victor.

The contest: Who had the widest thighs?

I wish I were joking. The depth of our depravity was revealed in our dorm room that evening. But the "winner" of the "widest thighs" contest couldn't be determined that easily. To this day, each of the participants (at least the ones who remember participating in this silly contest) remembers looking in that mirror and seeing herself as the biggest. Of course, we didn't *really* want to know whose upper legs were the fullest. *That would be insane.* But when someone complained that she had "wide thighs," everyone else chimed in that they had "wider" thighs . . . and before too long a contest was born.

This exemplifies fairly typical behavior for college-age girls, according to the *Journal of Eating Disorders*. A study they published in 2013 uncovered the prevalence of "fat talk," a phenomenon that takes place among young women when they try to outdo each other with self-deprecation. You know how it goes. One friend says, "Wow, look how my stomach sticks out." Then, to make her feel better, another responds by mentioning the part of her body she believes can rival her friend's perceived flaw. The study says we do this to make ourselves appear more humble.[1]

If you have matured beyond fat talk, don't worry. This same data likely calls out your habits, too. Once you are too old to debate who is the fattest of them all, you start squabbling over who has the most wrinkles. Social scientists refer to it as "old talk."[2] As a gym employee, there is no doubt in my mind as to the veracity of this study. If two women come into my class together, I will inevitably witness some version of one of these conversations. I have heard courtroom-caliber cases made as to who has the biggest bottom or most noticeable laugh lines.

All the time.

We need allies in our body image battle. But we *don't* need friends like this. We need other women we can trust who will honestly walk beside us through this issue without comparison. A commercial for the US Army from a few years ago showed the bravery and character of a soldier by calling him an "Army of One." But here's the truth. No one—whether on an actual battlefield or in day-to-day life—fights effectively as an army of one. God didn't set it up that way.

Ladies, we don't need more friends who will tell us that their thighs have more jiggle or to "embrace" our curves. No, we need women who will tell us the truth of the gospel as it relates to our physical bodies. We need women around us who boldly call us out when our focus drifts from serving and glorifying God to serving and glorifying ourselves.

My friend Anne (not her real name) stopped me after a kickboxing class one day. She said she really needed to talk to me. Anne and I have a lot in common (her husband works in ministry like mine), so I assumed she wanted to share a church-related struggle.

"Heather, I want to get implants. I mean, I really, really want to get them done. I know it's not technically wrong, but I feel like my heart is in the wrong place here, and it's probably not right for me. Help!" She was almost in tears because of her inner struggle between desire and rational thought. I told her that I understood. She confided that nursing just one baby had left her with what I'll just call a "depleted" supply. Having clocked four years of breastfeeding myself, I could relate.

Then I asked her why—why implants? Anne knows the truth. She understands the gospel, so she beat me to the punch line. "Oh, I know it won't make me happier. But every other friend I've asked says I should go for it, and I don't know what to make of that." Anne shared that, considering their current financial situation, augmentation surgery would be a ridiculous burden. But she just couldn't get the idea of "better" breasts out of her head.

My advice for Anne included the following three statements. First, God accepts you just the way you are—even when you can't accept yourself. Second, though there's nothing inherently sinful about getting surgery, it sounded like she felt convicted about it. So I encouraged her to listen to the Holy Spirit's leading. And finally, I said the following, "Anne, freedom is not going to come from deciding you love wearing an A cup. Freedom will not come from staring in the mirror and determining to love your body. Freedom is found in self-forgetfulness."

She cried a little and thanked me, relieved to have someone speak truth into her life.

I wish I could say I've always responded that way. But that simply wouldn't be true. I've done my fair share of pinching inches of flesh and declaring, "Mine's flabbier!" Or counting pimples and exclaiming, "Stop griping. I have more!"

My dream is for Christian women to relate to each other differently. Until our friendships move beyond superficial endorsements of our struggles, we battle alone. You may have 1,849 Facebook friends and as many Twitter and Instagram followers, but until you have one or two women in your life willing to listen to the heart behind your words, offer you grace, and show you how the gospel applies, you walk alone.

Do you want to know exactly what to say to a friend who says, "Look at how big my butt has gotten?" Here's your answer: "No matter what your size, you are already accepted and loved."

When she says, "I've gained so much weight. I just don't like myself anymore, and I don't know how he could like me, either." Just like I reminded Anne, you say, "Jesus thinks you were valuable enough to die for. He loves you no matter what number that tag says. He gives you grace. Give yourself grace, too. If you want to be healthier, I'll support you on your journey. But know you are already loved beyond measure."

We've gone through four steps you can take to find a new place of freedom in your body image battle. The fifth and final step encompasses ways for you to find victory and keep that freedom once attained, through help from others. The ways include companionship, community, and connection. (I know, I'm an alliteration nerd.)

Guess What? You're Normal

The private school where I attended junior and senior high had a fairly strict dress code. Skirts had to cover the knees, no obnoxious printed sayings or corporate logos on anything, pants couldn't be too tight, no jeans allowed. . . . *You get the idea.*

In eighth grade, I frequently had anxiety dreams where I would show up at school wearing the wrong clothing. In them, I would walk into the school, look down, and realize I was wearing Jordache jeans with an Izod shirt. (It was the 80s, and trust me, that was cool.) I would take four steps into the school's main lobby and then freeze in panic, knowing I'd have to pay the ultimate punishment for my grievous dress code error. I would be forced to wear my gym uniform all day long. My thirteen-year-old brain could think of nothing worse than wearing that totally uncool, not to mention unflattering, pair of red polyester shorts for an entire school day.

Sure, donning the uniform during gym was bad enough, but everyone in the class had it on. We were all unfortunate contestants in an anti-fashion show as we learned to serve a volleyball and toss a Frisbee. But sporting that outfit combo alone, outside of gym class, felt like death by humiliation.

Our struggles only compound when we try to handle them alone. The best way to be free from the body image struggles that bind us is to not battle solo. Just as confession to Christ begins the healing process, bringing our sins to the light with another person defeats the darkness. We find new freedom when we reveal our struggle to someone else. When we give words to what we are thinking, hearing, or suffering, we put ourselves on a new course.

What I love most about the little bit of friendly counseling I engage in as a pastor's wife is this one thing: letting women know they're not alone. In 1 Corinthians 10:13, we read that every temptation (sin) is common to all people. In other words, I can declare with absolute certainty that whatever you are struggling with, someone else has struggled with it, too. When I hear a woman pour her heart out—exposing the lies that the enemy has filled her mind with—and am able to say, "Yes, he says all those things to me, too. I know those lies. Does he also say this?" I get giddy. Often they answer in return, "Yes. But I didn't want to say that one out loud!"

I don't mean that I take joy in their pain. Rather, it thrills me to blow the enemy's cover. It makes me excited to help women find simple freedom in the fact that they are not alone. When I can play a role in helping another woman debunk one of the enemy's myths, I'm happy. I love seeing the relief on their faces. The "Okay, I guess I'm normal" reaction I read in their expression is better than any thank you.

Truthfully, every time I can strengthen a friend in this way, it also strengthens me. I, too, need the extra reminder. My heart is prone to doubt, and the extra evidence that the enemy, though cunning, is using the same old lies on all of us gives me new boldness. Or, as C. S. Lewis says in *The Four Loves*, "The typical expression of opening Friendship would be something like, 'What? You too? I thought I was the only one.'"[3]

The enemy wants to convince us that we're weird, unusual, the only one, and beyond hope. He wants us to think we're flawed and that no one else has our quirks, hang-ups, problems, or compulsions. No one else struggles not to go back to the freezer for a fifth taste of ice cream. No one else gives in to the temptation of all those candy bars at the grocery checkout line (and then hides the evidence in the garage trash can). No other woman considers how she could finish off the kids' cookies and replace them before anyone notices. He feeds us lies that condemn.

The deceiver tricks us into believing we're alone in the severity of our problems. Or, if others do struggle, it's significantly less than we do. So we keep quiet, lest anyone think we're freaks. We never find freedom because we are bound by shame and fear. We accept that we really are alone and that no one else would understand. We better not open our mouths or we'll risk humiliation.

Will You Be My Friend?

Maintaining close friendships as we move out of the school years and into careers, family, and the busyness of life grows increasingly difficult. Relationships deep enough to penetrate the surface issues of day-to-day life require intentionality.

I spent many years of my adult life without close friends. I falsely assumed I would be okay to bide my time until I found a husband, at which point I assumed I would have little need for close female companions. (I was way off on that one. No man will ever fully understand a woman, no matter how hard he tries. In the same way, my brain will never wrap around how a man can be telling the truth when he says he's thinking about "nothing.")

At age thirty-one, I moved across the country (from Washington, DC, to central California) with my brand-new husband. To my surprise, I was still frequently alone. I worked from home all day while he maintained an unpredictable military flight schedule. Pregnancy compounded my loneliness. Tired and emotional, the thought of making friends put me on tilt. I talked to a few ladies—mostly other pilots' wives in our squadron—but deep, heart-level discussions were rare. As my baby-producing years progressed, I found it easier to form friendships with other new moms. But, again, our conversations often centered on child-rearing.

When it was time for us to step into full-time ministry, advisors all but mandated I find some friends. They knew I would not survive the rigors of church planting without close confidants. Though the thought frightened me a bit, I also knew I needed to cultivate closer relationships with other women. It was hard—like putting four kids to bed in a hotel on the first night of vacation hard. I was busy. They were busy. It seemed like it would be too difficult to have the time required to develop any type of deep bond.

So I did something crazy. I asked someone to be my friend. I know, it all sounds so very first grade. But it's true. Another military wife named Karla had also relocated from California to Texas and lived just forty-five miles away. We arranged times to meet in the middle for play dates and dinner. Then I decided to make it formal. With all of the weirdness you'd expect, I humbly asked her one day, "Hey, will you be my friend?"

Her response was, "Wow, I'm honored. I'd love to be your friend." (Turns out it's a flattering question, not a scary one.) And you know what? Defining the relationship benefited both of us. She knew I wouldn't treat her struggles lightly. I held the same level of confidence that she would hear me out without judgment and offer either a Christ-centered perspective or prayer when she ran out of answers.

If you find yourself lacking friends, I encourage you to be bold and find some. Maybe you know someone casually who you think would make for a better friend if you had more time to spend together. Seek ways to build the relationship. Invite her to coffee. Ask her over with kids for a play date. See if she's been longing to try out that new cupcake shop, too.

Perhaps you have a different situation. Maybe you don't know where to start. What if there isn't anyone in your mental Rolodex who would qualify as potential friend material? For you, I recommend first finding community or a group of women where you could find an ally. If you don't attend church, that's a great first step. Many churches have small groups or specific groups for women that are already established. Other churches in your community may offer programs for specific groups of women such as MOPs (Mothers of Preschoolers), Moms Next, or Community Bible Study.

Community and Other Risky Ventures

I was raised on *Sesame Street*. I'm still a fan of Big Bird, Cookie Monster (of course, because I also have a thing for cookies), and even Oscar the Grouch (what a great reference to show my children the unpleasantness of their behavior when they're disagreeable). One game segment on the PBS show displayed a group of items and asked you to pick out which was different. A catchy song, "Which of these is not like the other?" accompanied the skills test. The pre-K version of me enjoyed the challenge of figuring out which item didn't belong.

When I join a new community, I feel like I'm a part of that *Sesame Street* game—the different one about to be axed off the screen as the outsider. When we planted our church a few years ago, I was forced into a community of people that I didn't choose. We were essentially alone when we started, so our group contained strangers and near strangers. I often felt like I had little in common with those around me. I struggled through years of discomfort, begging God to help me relate. Sometimes it felt impossible. Yet he was faithful to grow me. He answered my prayers—but not in the way I expected. Instead of sending me a community full of long-lost twin sisters, he helped me see how, beneath our surface differences, we had a whole lot in common.

If you also find community hard, relax. You are normal! Let me repeat that. You are not alone if you find it awkward or challenging to become part of a new group of people. The enemy feeds us this falsehood to keep us out of community with other believers. He tells us that we aren't like all the others. He shows us how different (or in some cases "off") they are and convinces us that we have nothing in common. He will do whatever it takes and say anything to keep us from connecting with a group of believers.

Community feels so risky. What if you open yourself up to this group and they don't accept you? What if you share something that they can't relate to, and they respond with blank stares and gaping mouths? What if you *really are* the only one who struggles? I'd encourage you, friend, not to believe these lies. More so, don't let them keep you from healthy community.

Want to verify this? Ask your pastor's wife. Chances are she's also witnessed or experienced the enemy's strategies at work. I watch people struggle to become integrated into the church and then use "We don't fit in" as their excuse for withdrawing. In most of these cases, my heart breaks because I see the self-sabotage involved.

The story often plays out like this: the individual or family becomes part of the group, and the ice begins to melt. Just as they start to participate, something comes up. Work gets busy or kids have sports conflicts. So they miss a few weeks of church and small group meetings. Before you know it, a month passes. Then two months. They no longer know what's going on. They haven't kept up with the study and start to feel disconnected from the group. They disengage further and further until they convince themselves they no longer are a part. Suddenly, they come to the conclusion that they don't fit in. Satan smiles.

This saddens me. It's often clear that their disconnection is not the fault of the community, but rather a byproduct of their choices. Becoming and remaining a part of community requires commitment, risk, and effort. Put community—church and group involvement—on your schedule first. Make this a priority. Sure, your church friends may understand better than the soccer coach why you can't make it. But misaligned priorities hurt you and your family in the long run. Your children will benefit more from parents who are involved in a healthy, Christ-centered community than they will from having perfect attendance on the soccer field (especially when they are only five years old and the teams don't keep score!).

I've also noticed how comparison keeps us out of healthy church community. The enemy tells women lies like, "You are too fat to be a part of that group." Or, "Your clothes aren't nice enough to fit in there. You better not go back." Lies. All lies. But they work way too often at keeping women away from deeper relationships with other believers. The concept of camaraderie abounds in the New Testament. You may have noticed that Jesus had a group of twelve guys he kept around all the time. Community is absolutely vital to our growth. We need people who say, "Hey, I struggle too," or people who can say back to us, "You know that's not actually true, right? You can't believe everything you think." If we don't have these people, then we miss out.

Weight Watchers, Alcoholics Anonymous, and CrossFit have all figured this out and use it to their advantage. One part of overcoming your struggle—whether you want to lose sixty pounds or stop drinking or start exercising regularly—is to join a group. When you hear other people say that they do the same compulsive thing you're ashamed of, you feel validated and empowered. Instead of feeling embarrassed, you feel normal. Facing the hurdles standing between you and your objective becomes easier.

I've watched Christian friends throw themselves into support groups of all types to help them accomplish their goals. In many cases, though, they neglect working through the heart level of the problem with other Christ-followers first. My friend Jenny (not her real name) joins Weight Watchers every single year to lose what is likely the same twenty-five pounds. Jenny's problem isn't her inability to stick to a diet plan. Nor does she lack willpower to avoid delicious foods. Jenny's problem rests in her heart.

As discussed in the previous steps, Jenny struggles with what she believes about food and God. Her participation in community helps her lose weight temporarily, but it's not a permanent solution because her community addresses only the symptoms of her struggle, not the cause.

Similarly, I have friends all over the country who are CrossFit addicts. I love CrossFit, and I commend their incredibly effective strategy—using community to help people reach their fitness goals.

But I'm concerned that many Christian friends who are devoted to their workout partners at CrossFit don't engage in the same level of connection to other believers. They may find great success in serving their bodies and strengthening themselves physically, but who will help them grow spiritually? Do they put the same level of effort into spiritual training as they invest in physical training? (See 1 Tim. 4:8. The Apostle Paul must have seen this happening in CrossFit Rome, too.)

Get involved in a community that will build you up spiritually. Many churches now participate in recovery programs like Celebrate Recovery. If your body image struggle consumes you or if you've struggled with a full-blown eating disorder, this makes a great place to find friends and support that will lead to greater freedom.

Some of us avoid community altogether because we worry too much about our reputation or what other people will think if we show them our areas of struggle. The book of Ecclesiastes approaches this topic in a helpful way. Read how King Solomon writes about the strength found in friends and community from Ecclesiastes 4:9–12:

> Two are better than one, because they have a good
> reward for their toil. For if they fall, one will lift up his
> fellow. But woe to him who is alone when he falls and
> has not another to lift him up! Again, if two lie together,
> they keep warm, but how can one keep warm alone?
> And though a man might prevail against one who is

alone, two will withstand him—a threefold cord is not quickly broken.

Community outweighs the risk. Those awkward first few weeks or months will pass. There may be messy times. Relationships are never perfect. But, invest your time, energy, and effort into authentic community, and you'll see how it helps you overcome your struggles.

A Case for Connecting with God

You might say I know my husband pretty well. After a decade together, I can tell you without hesitation his favorite foods, his clothing sizes, and his favorite sports teams. I know how he takes his coffee and the way he prefers his eggs.

Sometimes people from our church will ask me, "What does Pastor Eric think about this?" or "What would Pastor Eric say about that?" Unless it's something completely innocuous, I usually tell them to ask him directly. But the truth is, often I can predict his response. I know him and his default positions well enough that I could likely tell them his answer. I wish there was a game show for not-so-newlyweds to win money for predicting each other's answers.

What would happen, though, if I stopped talking to him today? If I told him we weren't going to communicate any more, how would that impact our relationship?

What I know about him probably wouldn't change. It's not likely he'll stop rooting for the Texas Rangers or decide he prefers poached eggs to scrambled. But our relationship would begin to change. The distance would become increasingly palpable. Misunderstandings would surface over issues that may have been overlooked if we were closer. I'd also expect our level of trust to diminish. I'd probably question how much he really loved me, and he would do the same. What about my ability to guess how he would respond on certain issues? After a year or so of not communicating, this talent would also wane. I'd become less certain as to how he would respond because of our lack of connection.

Some of us struggle because this exemplifies what has happened in our personal relationship with God. We know about him, and we've learned some facts about his character. We've memorized the stories and can effortlessly recite John 3:16. But we don't often communicate with the Father. We don't connect with him regularly.

Do you want to be free from the body image worry that consumes you? Spend more time with your Savior. Do you want to stop obsessing over calories, your obliques, or your cankles? Read more about how much Jesus loves you than you do about which exercises work best for toning your abs. *Please hear my heart.* I'm exasperated by the number of women, in bondage to body image, who tell me that they haven't opened their Bible in months or that they don't "have time" to pray.

My friend, I understand. But don't put repentance and re-prioritization on the back shelf. We can't afford to disconnect from our Savior. If you're like me, this may prove difficult. Since I was raised in the church and Christian schools, I find it easy to fool myself into thinking I already know enough. I wrestled with a complacent familiarity in my Christian walk that led me to believe I already knew God and that he "understood" when I was too busy to read his Word or pray.

He does give us grace and forgive us when this happens. Don't misunderstand me here. But it's not what he has for us. There's a better way. His design for our lives includes constant connection with him. Without connection, it's impossible to remember how much he loves us, and it becomes increasingly hard to trust his plan for our lives. The New Testament presents us with two choices. We can live with a kingdom mentality or a worldly mentality. James argues that it's near impossible to keep a kingdom mentality when you're disconnected from the King (James 4).

Let's be honest, the times we struggle most with our body image usually align with the times we find ourselves too absorbed in our culture. We listen to what TV, movies, magazine covers, books, or the makeup aisle shout at us. And if we don't combat that with ample connection to the King, who has a different message for us, those messages will win.

Make this your mandate. If you have time to check social media, you have time to read your Bible. You have just as many hours in a day as every other person on earth. Get creative if you must. Listen to the Bible in your car as you commute to work or drive your children around. Listen to sermon podcasts as you clean your house or fold laundry. Make a conscious decision to not check Pinterest or Instagram until you've opened your Bible app and read the chapter for the day. Put on your calendar—with a reminder—a designated ten-minute time slot to read your Bible and pray.

Connection to Christ will transform you. You need it. (Check out John 15:1–6 when you do the Heart Exercises below). You can't do it apart from him. You just can't.

You've reached step five: **Seek Help Through Companionship, Community, and Connection to God**. Use the Heart Exercises that follow to explore these topics.

Chapter Mirror

Through close friends, community, connection with Jesus, we continue to find victory and help for our body image battles. Sin thrives in the darkness of secrecy. Sharing our struggles with gospel-grounded friends in a gospel-centered community can set our souls free and help us defeat sin in our lives.

Heart Exercises

Read the passage from John 15:1–6.

1. How connected to Christ are you? Do you believe it's possible to bear fruit apart from this connection?

2. How does the level of your connection correlate to your struggle with body image?

3. Are you in community? In what ways do you think prioritizing community could help your struggle?

4. Do you have friends you can honestly share the secrets of your heart with? Why or why not?

Memory Verse: "Whoever walks with the wise becomes wise, but the companion of fools will suffer harm" (Prov. 13:20).

Notes

[1] Carolyn Black Becker, Phillippa Diedrichs, Glen Jankowski, and Chelsey Werchan, "I'm Not Just Fat, I'm Old: Has the Study of Body Image Overlooked 'Old Talk'?" *Journal of Eating Disorders* 1 no. 6. (February 2013), www.jeatdisord .com/content/1/1/6.

[2] Ibid.

[3] C. S. Lewis, *The Four Loves* (New York: Mariner Books, 1971), 106.

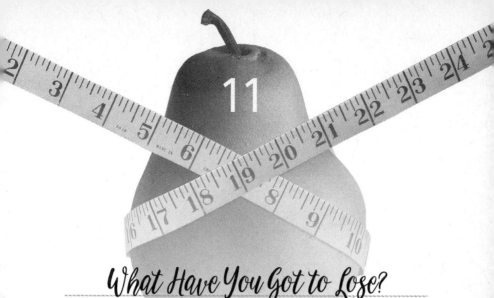

What Have You Got to Lose?

"The gospel is this: We are more sinful and flawed in ourselves than we ever dared believe, yet at the very same time we are more loved and accepted in Jesus Christ than we ever dared hope."

—TIM KELLER, *The Meaning of Marriage*

A British stylist named Gok Wan appeared on the *Today Show* as part of their "Love Your Selfie" series. The series garnered so much positive attention that they extended it to two full weeks of segments on women and our struggle with body image. Of all of the ideas I've heard about how to get comfortable with your cellulite, sagging, and rolls of flab, Gok's proved to be the strangest. His suggestion?

Get naked and look in the mirror.

What?

Gok asks women to come to his studio, undress in front of a full-length mirror, and just stare until they figure out how lovely they really are. Then he dresses them stylishly so they can feel even "better." My husband found it laugh-out-loud funny that a man would come up with "just get naked" as a solution for women who struggle. I found it strange that any women would consider it, let alone try it! Sounded like an April Fool's gag to me.

No, thank you!

You know that's not your answer. Our culture keeps drumming up new ideas to help you improve your body image. My question to you, friend, is do they work? Have they changed the pulse of your struggle at all? By now (unless you are one of those skip-to-the-back-of-the-book type of people like I am) you've read my answers. The only question remaining is, will you try it? If "loving the skin you're in" hasn't resolved this issue for you, then what do you have to lose?

My charge to you is to be brave. Boldly confess to your Heavenly Father where you've missed it and confidently go forth with a renewed identity in *whose* you are, not in who you are. Identify the ways beauty and comparison negatively impacted your relationship with your Father in heaven.

New diets will entice you. You'll be tempted to step onto that scale and say, "Forget it. I have to do something about this!" But let me encourage you to trust him fully to redeem your body image issues. Like Colossians 3:2 says, "Set your mind on things that are above." Meditate on his precepts instead of what your pre-baby abs looked like. Dwell in his great love for you instead of in the pit of despair over the twenty pounds that won't come off or that cellulite the cream can't seem to fade.

My prayer for you is to become consumed with a greater affection—that you will find Jesus satisfying in a way that even warm chocolate chip cookies can never match. As you engage in this book's five-step process—over and over again if necessary—I pray you will find satisfaction and peace in his love and approval. Alone.

Jesus is enough.

A Body Image Prayer

Dear Heavenly Father,

You know my heart and my struggle. You understand the wrestling match I'm in, trying to meet a cultural standard of beauty and knowing that in you is where my *true* value can be found. Today, please help me to remember Jesus's great sacrifice for me that had *nothing* to do with what I look like.

Help me to know that *I'm already enough with Jesus*—no matter what the scales or magazine covers say. Keep my focus this day on *you*, your kingdom, and your love and *off* my perceived body flaws. Remind me that my purpose for today is far greater than figuring out how I compare to *her* . . . or *her* . . . or *her*. Help me to aspire only to look and be more like *you*.

I need your strength, dear God. Please fill me with your spirit and empower me to fight this battle well today.

A Word to Those Struggling with Eating Disorders

By Jena Morrow, author of *Hollow: An Unpolished Tale*

First, you are to be commended for seeking resources like this one to guide and support you on your journey toward wholeness and health. The fact that you've picked up this book indicates that you have a desire to learn, grow, and change—and that cannot be said about everyone! Change can be scary and growth can be uncomfortable, but you are evidently not content to stay in bondage to the tyranny of perfectionism or to the self-hatred it can breed. Thank God for that!

If you are struggling with anorexia, bulimia, binge eating disorder, or any combination of these, it is essential that you take certain steps to ensure your safety as you work toward recovery. I have great hope for you and for all those in pursuit of recovery from eating disorders, and I believe that freedom is possible—and I also know that eating disorders carry the highest mortality rate of all other psychiatric disorders combined. Bottom line: you need a treatment team to ensure that you remain safely monitored while you work toward recovery.

I recommend, at a minimum, a physician and an individual therapist (preferably with some degree of knowledge or specialty in eating disorders), and these two professionals should have one another's contact information and releases of information, signed by you, in their files. Depending on your individual needs (as determined collaboratively and regularly assessed by you and your therapist), you may also benefit from including a psychiatrist, a dietician, and an eating disorder sponsor in your treatment team. Also, depending on the severity of your symptoms and your level of physical health, please be aware that a residential or partial hospitalization program may be advisable for a short time.

Finally, I want to encourage you, as one who has walked a path similar to yours, to persevere in your pursuit of a life free of the torture of eating disorders—no matter what. You will *not* "do recovery" perfectly, I assure you—but that's okay; after all, we cannot heal perfectionism *with* perfectionism! Just take it one day at a time, keep a firm grasp on the hand of our God who is an ever-present help in trouble, and do the next right thing. Better days are ahead . . . and hope is real!

About the Author

Heather Creekmore holds a Bachelor's degree in communication and a Master's degree in public policy. After almost a decade of part-time work in the fitness industry, Heather started a blog for Christian women who struggle with comparison and body image called "Compared to Who?"

Heather is married to Eric—an Acts 29 pastor and church planter in Texas—and mom to Zach, Katie, Trevor, and Drew. Before marriage and ministry, Heather spent twelve years working in political campaign management and for nonprofit causes. Her passion is to help women struggling with body image issues find God's grace and complete acceptance through the gospel (and to help strict grammarians loosen up just a bit).

Connect with Heather and join the movement of women ready to be free from comparison and body image struggles!

Blog: www.comparedtowho.me
Facebook: www.facebook.com/heathercreekmoreblog
Twitter: www.twitter.com/comparedtowho
Pinterest: www.pinterest.com/comparedtowho
Instagram: www.instagram.com/comparedtowho